ABC of
Kidney Disease

EDITED BY

David Goldsmith
Consultant Nephrologist, Guy's Hospital, London, UK

Satish Jayawardene
Consultant Nephrologist, King's College Hospital, London, UK

Penny Ackland
General Practitioner, Camberwell, London, UK

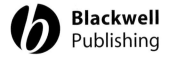
Blackwell Publishing

BMJ|Books

© Blackwell Publishing Ltd 2007

BMJ Books is an imprint of the BMJ Publishing Group, used under licence

Blackwell Publishing Inc., 350 Main Street, Malden, Massachusetts 02148-5020, USA
Blackwell Publishing Ltd, 9600 Garsington Road, Oxford OX4 2DQ, UK
Blackwell Publishing Asia Pty Ltd, 550 Swanston Street, Carlton, Victoria 3053, Australia

The right of the Author to be identified as the Author of the Work has been asserted in accordance with the Copyright, Designs and Patents Act 1988.

All rights reserved. No part of this publication may be reproduced, stored in a retrieval system, or transmitted, in any form or by any means, electronic, mechanical, photocopying, recording and/or otherwise, except as permitted by the UK Copyright, Designs and Patents Act 1988, without the prior written permission of the publisher.

First published 2007

1 2007

Library of Congress Cataloging-in-Publication Data

ABC of kidney disease / edited by David Goldsmith, Satish Jayawardene, and Penny Ackland.
     p. ; cm.
  ISBN-13: 978-1-4051-3675-4 (alk. paper)
  ISBN-10: 1-4051-3675-8 (alk. paper)
  1. Kidneys--Diseases. 2. Family medicine. I. Goldsmith, David, 1959- II. Jayawardene, Satish. III. Ackland, Penny.
  [DNLM: 1. Kidney Diseases. 2. Kidney Failure, Chronic. WJ 300 A134 2007]
  RC902.A333 2007
  616.6'1--dc22
                        2006103166

ISBN: 978-1-4051-3675-4

A catalogue record for this book is available from the British Library

Cover image of coloured computed tomography (CT) scan of a section through a whole healthy human kidney is courtesy of Alfred Pasieka / Science Photo Library

Set in 9.25 / 12 pt Minion by Sparks, Oxford – www.sparks.co.uk
Printed and bound at GraphyCems, Navarra, Spain

Commissioning Editor: Mary Banks
Associate Editor: Vicki Donald
Editorial Assistant: Victoria Pittman
Production Controller: Rachel Edwards

For further information on Blackwell Publishing, visit our website:
www.blackwellpublishing.com

The publisher's policy is to use permanent paper from mills that operate a sustainable forestry policy, and which has been manufactured from pulp processed using acid-free and elementary chlorine-free practices. Furthermore, the publisher ensures that the text paper and cover board used have met acceptable environmental accreditation standards.

Blackwell Publishing makes no representation, express or implied, that the drug dosages in this book are correct. Readers must therefore always check that any product mentioned in this publication is used in accordance with the prescribing information prepared by the manufacturers. The author and the publishers do not accept responsibility or legal liability for any errors in the text or for the misuse or misapplication of material in this book.

Contents

Contributors

Penny Ackland

General Practitioner, Camberwell, London, UK

Behdad Afzali

Specialist Registrar Nephrology and MRC Clinical Research Fellow, Department of Nephrology and Transplantation, Guy's Hospital, London, UK

Aminu Kasarawa Bello

Clinical Research Fellow, Sheffield Kidney Institute, Sheffield Teaching Hospitals NHS Trust, Sheffield, UK

Richard Burden

Consultant Nephrologist, Nottingham City Hospital, Nottingham, UK

James O Burton

Clinical Research Fellow, Department of Renal Medicine, Derby City Hospital, Derby, UK

Frances Coldstream

Consultant Nurse in Predialysis Management, Guy's and St Thomas' NHS Foundation Trust, London, UK

Mohsen El Kossi

Specialist Registrar Renal and General Medicine, Sheffield Kidney Institute, Sheffield Teaching Hospitals NHS Trust, Sheffield, UK

A Meguid El Nahas

Professor of Nephrology, Sheffield Kidney Institute, University of Sheffield, Sheffield, UK

John Feehally

Consultant Nephrologist, The John Walls Renal Unit, Leicester General Hospital, Leicester, UK

Sean Gallagher

Senior House Officer, Renal Medicine, Guy's Hospital, London, UK

David Goldsmith

Consultant Nephrologist, Guy's Hospital, London, UK

Rizwan Hamer

Specialist Registrar, Renal Unit, Birmingham Heartlands Hospital, Birmingham, UK

Ming He

Clinical Fellow in Transplant Surgery, Renal Unit, Guy's Hospital, London, UK

Rachel Hilton

Consultant Nephrologist, Guy's Hospital, London, UK

Richard Hull

Specialist Registrar Nephrology, Guy's Hospital, London, UK

Satish Jayawardene

Consultant Nephrologist, King's College Hospital, London, UK

Philip Kalra

Consultant Nephrologist and Honorary Senior Lecturer, Hope Hospital, Salford, UK

Douglas Maclean

Renal Pharmacist, Guy's Hospital, London, UK

Christopher W McIntyre

Reader in Vascular Medicine, Department of Renal Medicine, Derby City Hospital, Derby, UK

Donal O'Donoghue

Consultant Renal Physician, Hope Hospital, Salford, UK
National Clinical Director for Renal Services

Christopher Reid

Consultant Paediatric Nephrologist, Evelina Children's Hospital, St Thomas' Hospital, London, UK

Neil S Sheerin

Clinical Senior Lecturer, King's College, London, UK; Honorary Consultant, Department of Nephrology and Transplantation, Guy's Hospital, London, UK

John Taylor

Consultant Transplant Surgeon, Department of Renal Medicine and Transplantation, Guy's Hospital, London, UK

Judy Taylor

Consultant Paediatric Nephrologist, Evelina Children's Hospital, St Thomas' Hospital, London, UK

Charlie Tomson

Consultant Nephrologist, Southmead Hospital, Bristol, UK

Preface

Why a book on *kidney disease*? A reasonable question once, but no more. From its rather austere, academic origins focusing on renal tubular physiology, the awkward child 'nephrology' has now matured into the confident adult 'kidney disease' of a much greater relevance to the tens of thousands of healthcare workers involved in the complicated and sometimes frustrating business of preventing and curing ill-health.

Even the word 'kidney', so long shunned in favour of 'renal' or 'nephrological' as a partner for the word 'disease', has a new context now – the International Society of Nephrology (well, no one is perfect), the European Renal Association (ditto) and many other organizations have designated the second Thursday in every March as 'World Kidney Day'.

The practice of renal replacement therapy (which describes dialysis and renal transplantation) started in earnest in the 1960s, and in that decade where the star of technological advance burnt so brightly, most of the important technological advances in the provision of dialysis were made. Initially, dialysis was seen as an acute intervention and as a bridge to renal recovery or to renal transplantation. Significant numbers of patients started to undergo organ transplantation at around this time, again as the result of technological advances in immunosuppression – the use of steroids and azathioprine.

The evolution of the treatment of kidney disorders thereafter has been slower, though far more people are now undergoing long-term dialysis than could ever have been envisaged by the 'founding fathers' in both renal medicine and government. The cost of long-term provision of renal support has taxed many healthcare systems, but few so cruelly as the National Health Service, which for decades provided a second-rate service palpably inferior to what was available in Europe and particularly North America (not a unique failing as we can see from international comparisons with cardiac and also cancer services). Under these difficult circumstances the fact that kidney medicine and surgery not only survived, but flourished in the UK, is a testament to the dedication and zeal of those early pioneers.

With greater funding in recent years, the early embrace of independent-sector service provision, and most recently, a National Service Framework (2005) and a National Clinical Director (2007), we can now envisage not only the continuation of the significant 'catching up' with other European countries that began more than a decade ago, but also being able to rise to the challenges of the next few decades, chief amongst which are the early detection of chronic kidney problems and the prevention of both kidney decline and cardiovascular disease at this early stage.

This book is not a comprehensive, exhaustive, compendium of all things renal. It is, deliberately, a book which we hope will explain, to a sensible and practical level, acute and chronic kidney ailments, dialysis and renal transplantation. It is 'pitched' at hospital and general practitioners, and wider multi-disciplinary healthcare workers, and therefore does not assume expertise before the book is opened. This is, by design, a contrast with much larger, multi-author, multi-volume tomes gathering dust on library shelves, in which one can find the most minute descriptions of every one of the myriad ways in which the kidney can suffer from intrinsic as well as systemic diseases.

We want to feel that this book will be consulted daily, be accessible, approachable and act as one of the ways in which kidney disease can be de-mystified. If we have succeeded in this aim, it will be as a result of the excellent contributions of many chapter authors, the publishers and the helpful reviewers, all of whom we, the editors, most heartily thank for their efforts.

Acknowledgement

Figures 1.2, 1.3, 1.6, 4.4, 4.5, 4.6, 5.1, 5.2, 5.3, 5.4, 5.5, 5.6, 6.1, 6.3, 6.4, 7.3, 7.4, 7.5, 7.8, 7.9, 7.10, 11.2, 11.7, 11.8, 11.11, 11.12, 11.13 and 11.14 are reproduced with permission from Pattison J *et al.* (2004) *A Colour Handbook of Renal Medicine*. Manson Publishing Ltd: London.

CHAPTER 1

Diagnostic Tests in Chronic Kidney Disease

Behdad Afzali, Satish Jayawardene, David Goldsmith

OVERVIEW

- Urinary protein excretion of < 150 mg/day is normal (~30 mg of this is albumin and about 70–100 mg is Tamm-Horsfall (muco)protein, derived from the proximal renal tubule). Protein excretion can rise transiently with fever, acute illness, UTI and orthostatically. In pregnancy, the upper limit of normal protein excretion is around 300 mg/day. Persistent elevation of albumin excretion (microalbuminuria) and other proteins can indicate renal or systemic illness.

- Repeat positive dipstick tests for blood and protein in the urine two or three times to ensure the findings are persistent.

- Microalbuminuria is an early sign of renal and cardiovascular dysfunction with adverse prognostic significance.

- Microscopic haematuria is present in around 4% of the adult population – of whom at least 50% have glomerular disease.

- If initial GFR is normal, and proteinuria is absent, progressive loss of GFR amongst those people with microscopic haematuria of renal origin is rare, although long-term (and usually community-based) follow-up is still recommended.

- Adults 50 years old or more should undergo cystoscopy if they have microscopic haematuria (MH).

- Any patient with MH who has abnormal renal function, proteinuria, hypertension and a normal cystoscopy, should be referred to a nephrologist.

- Blood pressure control, reduction of proteinuria and cholesterol reduction are all useful therapeutic manoeuvres in those with renal causes of MH.

- All MH patients should have long-term follow-up of their renal function and blood pressure (this can, and often should be, community-based).

- Renal function is measured using creatinine, and this is now routinely converted into an estimated glomerular filtration rate (eGFR) value quickly and easily.

- The most common imaging technique now used for the kidney is the renal ultrasound, which can detect size, shape, symmetry of kidneys, and presence of tumour, stone or renal obstruction.

Table 1.1 Signs and symptoms of chronic kidney disease

Symptoms	Signs
Tiredness	Pallor
Anorexia	Leuconychia
Nausea and vomiting	Peripheral oedema
Itching	Pleural effusion
Nocturia, frequency, oliguria	Pulmonary oedema
Haematuria	Raised blood pressure
Frothy urine	
Loin pain	

Symptoms of chronic kidney disease (CKD) are often non-specific (Table 1.1). Clinical signs (of CKD, or of systemic diseases or syndromes) may be present and recognised early on in the natural history of kidney disease but more often, both symptoms and signs are only present and recognized very late – sometimes too late to permit effective treatment in time to prepare for dialysis. However the most commonly performed test of renal function – plasma creatinine – is typically performed in every hospital inpatient and as part of investigations or screening during many GP surgery or hospital clinic outpatient episodes.

Unlike 'angina' or 'chronic obstructive airways disease' where a history can be revealing (e.g. walking distance; cough) there is little that is quantifiable about CKD severity without blood and/or urine testing.

This is why serendipitous discovery of kidney problems (haematuria, proteinuria, structural abnormalities on kidney imaging, or loss of kidney function) is a common 'presentation'. A full understanding of what these abnormalities mean and a clear guide to 'what to do next' are particularly needed in kidney medicine, and filling this gap is one of the aims of this book.

Correct use and interpretation of urine dipsticks and plasma creatinine values (by far the commonest tests used for screening and identification of kidney disease) is the main focus of this chapter. Renal imaging and renal biopsy will also be described briefly.

Urine testing

Urinalysis is a basic test for the presence and severity of kidney disease. Testing urine during the menstrual period in women, and within 2–3 days of heavy strenuous exercise in both genders, should be avoided to avoid contamination or artefacts. Fresh 'mid-stream' urine is best, again to reduce accidental contamination. Refrigeration of urine at temperatures from +2 to +8°C assists preservation. Specimens that have languished in an overstretched hospital laboratory specimen reception area, before eventually undergoing analysis, will rarely reveal all of the potential information that could have been gained.

Table 1.2 The main causes of differently coloured urine

Pink–red–brown–black	Yellow–brown	Blue–green
Gross haematuria (e.g. bladder or renal tumour; IgA nephropathy)	**Jaundice**	**Drugs**: triamterene
Haemoglobinuria (e.g. drug reaction)	**Drugs**: chloroquine, nitrofurantoin	**Dyes**: methylene blue
Myoglobinuria (e.g. rhabdomyolysis)		
Acute intermittent porphyria		
Alkaptonuria		
Drugs: phenytoin, rifampicin (red); metronidazole, methyldopa (darkening on standing)		
Foods: beetroot, blackberries		

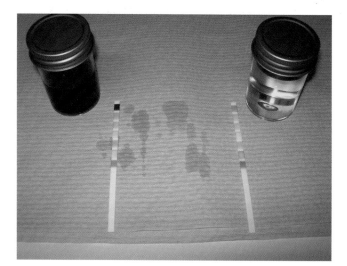

Figure 1.1 Urine dipstick – the urine on the right is normal and the colours of all of the squares on the urine dipstick are normal/negative. The urine on the left is from someone with acute glomerulonephritis, looks pink-brown macroscopically, and has maximal blood and protein on the dipstick.

Table 1.3 The main causes of false negative and positive testing from use of urine dipsticks

Test	False positive	False negative
Haemoglobin	Myoglobin	Ascorbic acid
	Microbial peroxidases	Delayed examination
Proteinuria	Very alkaline urine (pH 9)	Tubular proteins
	Chlorhexidine	Immunoglobulin light chains
		Globulins
Glucose	Oxidizing detergents	UTI
		Ascorbic acid

Discounting contamination from menstrual – or other – bleeding, and exercise-induced haematuria and proteinuria

Changes in urine colour are usually noticed by patients. Table 1.2 shows the main causes of different coloured urine. For information concerning changes in urine turbidity, odour and other physical characteristics consult a reference source.

Chemical parameters of the urine that can be detected using dipsticks include urine pH, haemoglobin, glucose, protein, leucocyte esterase, nitrites and ketones. Figure 1.1 shows the dipstick in its 'dry'

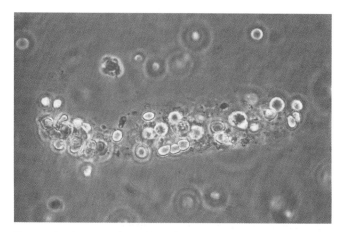

Figure 1.2 Microscopy of centrifuged fresh urine. There is a red cell cast (protein skeleton with incorporated red blood cells). This is characteristic of acute glomerulonephritis.

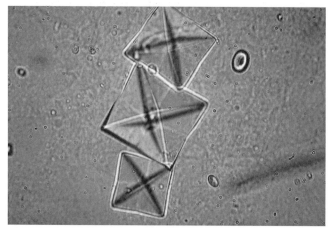

Figure 1.3 Crystalluria.

state, and also an example of a positive test. Table 1.3 shows the main false negative and false positive results that can interfere with correct interpretation.

Urine microscopy can only add useful information to urinalysis when there is a reliable methodology for collection, storage and analysis. This is often lacking, even in hospitals. Early morning urine is best, with rapid sample centrifugation. Under ideal circumstances *cells* (erythrocytes, leucocytes, renal tubular cells and urinary epithelial cells), *casts* (cylinders of proteinaceous matrix), *crystals*, *lipids* and *organisms* can be reliably identified where present in urine. Figure 1.2 shows a red cell cast in urine (indicative of acute renal inflammation). Figure 1.3 shows urinary crystals.

Microscopic haematuria (MH)

Definition and background
In healthy people red blood cells (rbc) are not present in the urine in >95% of cases. Large amounts of rbc make the urine pink or red.

MH is commonly defined as the presence of greater than two rbcs per high power field in a centrifuged urine sediment. It is seen in 3–6% of the normal population, and in 5–10% of those relatives of kidney patients who undergo screening for potential kidney donation.

MH can be an incidental finding of no prognostic importance, or the first sign of intrinsic renal disease, or urological malignancy. It always requires assessment, and most often also requires referral to a kidney specialist or to a urologist.

Clinical features

The finding of MH is usually as a result of routine medical examination for employment, insurance or GP-registration purposes in an otherwise apparently healthy adult. Initially, therefore, MH is an issue for primary healthcare workers. The goal of an assessment is to understand whether:

1 there are any clues available from the patient's history, his/her family history, or from examination, to point to a particular diagnosis, e.g. connective tissue disease, sickle cell disease;
2 the haematuria is transient or persistent;
3 there is any evidence of renal disease, e.g. abnormal renal function, accompanying proteinuria, raised blood pressure (BP);
4 the haematuria represents glomerular (i.e. from the kidney) or extra-glomerular (urological) bleeding.

Investigations

Typically the full evaluation of MH requires hospital-based investigations. Box 1.1 lists these in a logical order.

- *Urine microscopy and culture* should also be undertaken. The presence of dysmorphic red cells in the urine increases the possibility of intrinsic/parenchymal kidney disease as opposed to urological disease. This can only be ascertained in a specialist laboratory.
- *Renal structure* can be assessed with a renal ultrasound scan (this can show stones, cysts and tumours). A plain abdominal film will show radio-opaque renal, ureteric or bladder calculi. Renal function should be assessed by measurement of plasma biochemistry and es-

---

Box 1.1 **Investigations required for the work-up of patients with microscopic haematuria**

- Protein:creatinine ratio in fresh urine (if present on urinary dipstick testing)
- Urine microscopy and culture
- Plasma biochemistry and eGFR
- Autoantibody screen e.g. anti-nuclear antibody (ANA) and anti-neutrophil cytoplasmic antibody (ANCA) and complement levels (C3 and C4)
- Renal ultrasound
- Renal CT/MRI (in certain cases)
- Cystoscopy for adults > 50 years of age
- Renal biopsy in certain circumstances

---

timated glomerular filtration rate (eGFR). In addition, proteinuria should be looked for by dipstick analysis of the urine and, if present, a protein/creatinine ratio measured. Proteinuria >0.5 g/24 h (protein:creatinine ratio > 50) suggests glomerular disease and a referral to a kidney specialist is warranted for MH with significant proteinuria, raised BP or abnormal renal function.

Management

Any patient who presents with persistent microscopic haematuria over the age of 50 should be referred to a urologist. A renal ultrasound and a flexible cystoscopy to exclude urological cancer would normally be undertaken.

Any patient who has abnormal renal function, proteinuria, hypertension and a normal cystoscopy should be referred to a kidney specialist.

Renal biopsy is required to establish a diagnosis with absolute certainty in most cases of 'renal haematuria'. Those patients who have renal impairment, heavy proteinuria, hypertension, positive autoantibodies, low complement levels or have a family history of renal disease should undergo a renal biopsy.

Prognosis

The prognosis for most patients with asymptomatic MH without urological malignancy and no evidence of intrinsic renal disease is very good. It is beyond the scope of this chapter to discuss the prognosis of all the causes of microscopic haematuria, as listed in Table 1.4. However, some general observations apply for those patients in whom there is no structural cause for microscopic haematuria and bleeding is glomerular, and these are given below.

In the presence of impaired renal function, it is mandatory to try to achieve blood pressure control (< 130/80 mmHg) and reduction of microalbuminuria or proteinuria (if present). Angiotensin converting enzyme (ACE) inhibitors or angiotensin II receptor blockers (ARBs) are useful agents as they achieve both of these desired effects. It is very important to recheck plasma creatinine and potassium about 7–14 days after starting ACE or ARB, and regularly thereafter – an increase of > 20% in plasma creatinine from baseline, or similar fall in eGFR, or a rise of plasma potassium to exceed 5.5 mmol/L, should occasion recall to consider abandoning the drugs or reducing the dose, further investigations, and dietary advice for potassium restriction if relevant.

It is important that these patients, whether monitored in the community or at a hospital-based clinic, have their urine tested, BP measured and renal function monitored regularly. If not under renal specialist follow-up, the development of hypertension, proteinuria or deterioration in renal function are all indications for re-referral to a specialist unit (see Chapter 2).

Table 1.4 Causes of microscopic haematuria

Renal causes	Systemic causes	Miscellaneous and urological causes
IgA nephropathy	Systemic lupus erythematosus	Cystic diseases of the kidney
Thin basement membrane disease	Henoch–Schönlein purpura	Papillary necrosis
Alport's syndrome		Urothelial tumours
Focal segmental glomerulosclerosis		Renal and bladder stones
Membranoproliferative glomerulonephritis		Exercise-induced haematuria
Post-infectious glomerulonephritis		

Table 1.5 Equivalent ranges for urinary protein loss

	Urine dipstick	Albumin excretion rate (AER) (µg/min ; mg/24 h)		Urinary albumin:creatinine ratio (mg/mmol)	Protein (mg)/ creatinine (mmol)	Urinary protein (mg/24 h)
Normal	0	6–20 ;	10–30	<2.5 (m) <3.5 (w)	<15	<150
Microalbuminuria	0	>20–200 ;	30–300	>2.5 (m) >3.5 (w)	<15	<150
'Trace' proteinuria	Trace	>200 ;	>300	15–29	15–29	150–299
Proteinuria	+, ++	N/A	N/A	N/A	30–350	300–3500
Nephrotic	+++	N/A	N/A	N/A	>350	>3.5 g

m: men; w: women.

Microalbuminuria (MAU) and Proteinuria (P)

Protein is normally present in urine in small quantities. Tubular proteins (e.g. Tamm-Horsfall) and low amounts of albumin can be detected in healthy people. Microalbuminuria (MAU) refers to the presence of elevated urinary albumin concentrations (currently between lower and upper limits, see Table 1.5); MAU is a sign of either systemic or renal malfunction.

MAU is measured by quantitative immunoassay – and is an important first and early sign of many renal conditions, particularly diabetic renal disease and other glomerulopathies. It is also strongly associated with adverse cardiovascular outcomes. Around 10% of the population can be shown to have persistent MAU. For confirmation, two out of three consecutive analyses should show MAU in the same three-month period.

UAER (urinary albumin excretion rate) – in a healthy population the normal range for UAER is 1.5–20 µg/min. UAER increases with strenuous exercise, high protein diet, pregnancy and urinary tract infections. Daytime UAER is 25% higher than at night (so for daytime urine, an upper normal limit of 30 µg/min is often used). Overnight timed collections can be performed (and microalbuminuric range is an overnight UAER of 20–200 µg/min), but for unselected population screening the albumin:creatinine ratio (ACR) in early morning urine is preferable. An ACR of > 2 predicts a UAER of > 30 µg/min with a high sensitivity.

Increasingly favoured as a screening tool is the urinary protein-creatinine ratio (**PCR**). This is best done on 'spot' early morning urine samples (as renal protein excretion has a diurnal rhythm - see below). This is now preferable to relying on 24 hour urine collections (which are rarely thus). There is an inherent assumption in using PCR that urinary creatinine concentration is 10 mmol/L (in practice it can range from 5–30) but this is of little practical importance for its use as a screening tool. A PCR of 100 mg/mmoL corresponds roughly with 1 gram per litre of proteinuria.

One question often asked is how to 'convert' an ACR to a PCR. At low levels of proteinuria (< 1 g/day), a rough conversion is that doubling the ACR will give you the PCR. At proteinuria excretion rates of > 1 g/day, the relationship is more accurately represented by $1.3 \times ACR = PCR$.

Table 1.5 attempts to display all of the different ways to express urinary protein to allow for comparisons between methods.

Please note that the normal range for protein excetion in pregnancy is up to 300 mg/day, with clinical significance (pre-eclampsia or renal disease) being more likely once 500 mg or more is excreted per day. See Chapter 6, page 31.

Tests of kidney function

The kidney has exocrine and endocrine functions. The most important function to assess however is renal excretory capacity which we measure as *glomerular filtration rate* (GFR). Each kidney has about 1 million nephrons and the measured GFR is the composite function of all nephrons in both kidneys and conceptually it can be understood as the (virtual) clearance of a substance from a volume of plasma into the urine per unit of time. The substance can be endogenous (creatinine, cystatin C) or exogenous (inulin, iohexol, iothalamate, ^{51}Cr-EDTA, ^{99m}Tc-DTPA). The ideal substance does not exist – ideal characteristics being free filtration across the glomerulus, neither reabsorption from nor excretion into renal tubules, in a steady state concentration in plasma, and easily and reliably measured. Despite creatinine failing several of these criteria it is universally used, and we shall concentrate on interpreting creatinine concentration in urine and blood as it aids derivation of GFR.

The basic anatomy of the kidney and the anatomy and basic physiology of the 'nephron' (the functional component of the kidney), are shown in Figure 4.1 (page 15).

Table 1.6 shows the different ways in which both plasma urea and plasma creatinine may be 'artefactually' elevated or reduced which

Table 1.6 Problems with sole reliance on plasma concentrations of urea and creatinine to determine renal function

Factors independent of renal function that can affect plasma urea	Factors independent of renal function that can affect plasma creatinine	Other factors that can affect interpretation of plasma creatinine values
Hydration	Diet (meat)	Use of Jaffe reaction in laboratories:
Burns	Creatine supplements (e.g. body	interference by glucose, ascorbate,
Steroids	builders)	acetoacetate
Diuretics	Age	Use of enzymatic reaction in laboratories:
Liver disease	Body habitus	interference by ethamsylate or flucytosine
Diet (protein)	Race	

Distribution of creatinine according to GFR in stage 3 CKD

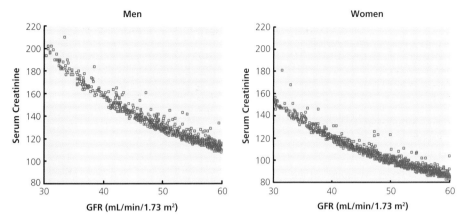

Figure 1.4 Relationship between plasma creatinine and glomerular filtration rate (GFR).

$$\text{GFR (mL/min/1.73 m}^2) = 186 \times [\text{serum creatinine (μmol/L)} \times 0.011312]{-}1.154 \times [\text{age}]{-}0.203 \times [1.212 \text{ if black}] \times [0.742 \text{ if female}]$$

Figure 1.5 Four-variable MDRD equation for eGFR.

can lead to misunderstanding and miscalculation of renal function. Creatinine is measured by two quite different techniques in the laboratory – one, the Jaffe reaction, relies on creatinine reacting with an alkaline picrate solution but is not specific for creatinine (e.g. cephalosporins, acetoacetate and ascorbate), while the other, the enzymatic method, is more accurate. Eventually isotope-dilution mass spectroscopy (IDMS) may render both of these variously flawed techniques redundant, either by direct substitution of method or by allowing IDMS-traceable creatinine values to be reported.

Creatinine is produced at an almost constant rate from muscle-derived creatine and phosphocreatine. However, as can be seen from Fig. 1.4 it is an insensitive marker of early loss of renal function (fall in GFR), and as renal function declines there is correspondingly more tubular creatinine secretion. It varies with diet, gender, disease state and muscle mass.

eGFR

The manipulation of plasma creatinine to derive a rapid estimation of creatinine clearance is very useful clinically, and is now formally recommended (as of April 2006 – see Chapters 2 and 3) to aid appropriate identification and referral of patients with CKD. There are several formulaic ways of doing this, and the formula that has been adopted in the UK, USA and many countries is the four-variable Modified Diet in Renal Disease (MDRD) formula (Fig. 1.5 and Chapter 2), but it must be appreciated that this formula may not be (as) accurate in ethnic minority patients, in the elderly, in pregnant women, the malnourished, amputees, or in children under 16 years of age.

Useful though deriving a value for GFR is, the value derived using the MDRD formula is only an *estimate* whose accuracy diminishes as GFR exceeds 60 mL/min, and values should therefore be viewed as having significant error margins rather than being precise. Values can only properly be used when renal function is in 'steady state', i.e. not in acute renal failure. It is unwise to rely exclusively on the formula between eGFR 60 and 89 mL/min (CKD stage 2) because of its shortcomings, while values > 90 mL/min should be reported thus (i.e. not as a precise figure). There is an urgent unmet need for better markers, and better formulae.

Formal nuclear medicine or research laboratory-derived measures of GFR are expensive, time-consuming and largely (and increasingly) confined to research studies.

Renal imaging

There is a wide range of imaging techniques available to localize and interrogate the kidneys. Table 1.7 gives the preferred methods for a range of conditions. Intravascular contrast studies are still used, though ultrasound has replaced most IVU/IVP examinations. Low osmolar non-ionic agents are less nephrotoxic and better tolerated. Reactions to contrast agents can be severe, though rarely life-threatening. In addition, renal impairment (usually mild and reversible, sometimes severe and irreversible) can be seen after the use of intravenous contrast. In patients with a plasma creatinine > 130 μmol/L (eGFR < 60 mL/min), thought must be given to the wisdom of the investigation. Pre-existing renal impairment, advanced age, diabetes and diuretic use or dehydration significantly increase the risk of contrast-induced nephropathy. The mainstay of prevention is understanding the risk, avoiding dehydration (by judiciously hydrating patients and promoting urine flow) using saline or 0.45% sodium bicarbonate. The dopamine agonist fenoldopam and the anti-oxidant *N*-acetylcysteine have both been proposed as protective agents; oral *N*-acetylcysteine has been widely assessed with conflicting results and its role remains uncertain. However, it is an inexpensive agent

Table 1.7 Renal imaging techniques and their main indications/applications

Condition	Technique
Renal failure	Ultrasound
Proteinuria/nephrotic syndrome	Ultrasound
Renal artery stenosis	MRA
Renal stones	Plain abdominal film
	Non-contrast CT
Renal infection	Ultrasound or CT abdomen
Retroperitoneal fibrosis	CT abdomen

MRA; magnetic resonance angiogram.

Box 1.2 **Reasons for enlarged or shrunken kidneys on renal imaging**

Large kidneys – symmetrical
Diabetes
Acromegaly
Amyloidosis
Lymphoma

Large kidney – asymmetrical
Compensatory hypertrophy (eg. secondary to nephrecotmy)
Renal vein thrombosis

Large kidneys –irregular outline
Polycystic kidney disease
Other multicystic disease

Small kidneys – symmetrical
Chronic kidney disease
Bilateral renal artery stenosis
Bilateral hypoplasia

Small kidney – unilateral
Renal artery stenosis
Unilateral hypoplasia
Scarring from reflux nephropathy

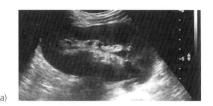
(a)

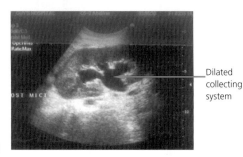
(b)

Dilated collecting system

Figure 1.6 (a) Ultrasound appearance of a normal kidney - dark areas represent renal cortex, and the central white area is the renal pelvis and collecting system. (b) An obstructed kidney, which shows in its centre a severely dilated renal pelvis and calyces (containing urine which is 'dark' on ultrasound).

without significant side-effects and its use in clinical practice may not therefore be inappropriate.

A comprehensive review of all imaging techniques is beyond the scope of this chapter. We shall concentrate on *ultrasound* imaging as this is by far the most often used for screening and investigation. Reference to radionuclide imaging, and IVU/IVP is made in Chapter 8. Renal size is usually in proportion to body height, and normally lies between 9 and 12 cm. Box 1.2 shows reasons for enlarged or shrunken kidneys. The *echo-consistency* of the renal cortex is reduced compared to medulla and the collecting system. In adults the loss of this 'cortico-medullary differentiation' is a sensitive but non-specific marker of CKD. Apart from renal size and cortico-medullary differentiation, the other significant abnormalities reported by ultrasound include the presence of cysts (simple, complex), solid lesions, and urinary obstruction. Figure 1.6 shows a normal kidney (a) and an obstructed kidney (b). Examination of the bladder and prostate is usually undertaken alongside scanning of native (or transplanted) kidneys.

Renal angiography and other techniques relevant to renal blood vessels are covered in Chapter 5. Radionuclide imaging is used for renal scars and urinary reflux, which is also mentioned in part in Chapter 8.

Renal biopsy

A renal biopsy is undertaken to investigate and diagnose renal disease in native and transplanted kidneys. Table 1.8 shows the main indications, contra-indications, and complications of this test. It is a highly specialized investigation, which should only be performed after careful consideration of the risk to benefit ratio, and with the close support of experienced imaging and renal histopathological teams.

Further reading

Van de Wal RM, Voors AA, Gansevoort RT. (2006) Urinary albumin excretion and the renin-angiotensin system in cardiovascular risk management. *Expert Opin Pharmacother*; **7**(18):2505–20.
NHS Information National Library for Kidney Disease, www.library.nhs.uk/kidney
www.renal.org/eGFR/haematuria.html
www.renal.org/eGFR/proteinuria.html
www.renal.org/eGFR/refer.html

Table 1.8 Indications for renal biopsy

Indications	Contra-indications	Complications
Nephrotic syndrome	Multiple renal cysts	Pain
Systemic disease with proteinuria or kidney failure	Solitary kidney (relative)	Bleeding – haematoma, haematuria (significant in <5%)
Acute renal failure	Acute pyelonephritis/abscess	
Proteinuria (PCR >50–100)	Renal neoplasm	Other organ biopsied (e.g. colon, spleen, liver)
Proteinuria and micro/macro-haematuria	Uncontrolled blood pressure	Arterio-venous fistula (0.1%)
Unexplained chronic renal failure	Abnormal blood clotting	Nephrectomy (<0.1%)
Transplanted kidney	Morbid obesity (relative)	Death (<0.01%)
	Inability to consent, or to comply with instructions	

CHAPTER 2

Screening and Early Intervention in Chronic Kidney Disease

Richard Burden, Charlie Tomson

OVERVIEW

- Studies suggest around 10% of the population has CKD.
- CKD is more common amongst the elderly, Afro-Caribbean and South Asian populations, and in those with hypertension or diabetes.
- The most common cause of established renal failure is diabetes mellitus.
- Late referral of patients reaching established renal failure is associated with increased morbidity and mortality.
- The greatest risk for patients with early CKD is of premature cardiovascular disease.
- Treating cardiovascular risk factors also slows progression of CKD.
- Selective screening for markers of CKD is recommended.
- Specialist referral is not necessary for the majority of patients with CKD.
- Microalbuminuria can be reduced or even reversed by the use of angiotensin-converting enzyme inhibitors and/or angiotensin receptor blockers.
- Integrated community-based chronic disease management is best practice for patients with CKD who are not under specialist care.

Despite mounting evidence that progressive loss of kidney function can be slowed, or even prevented, by timely treatment, the incidence of established renal failure continues to rise. Even in countries with comprehensive healthcare systems, many patients reaching established renal failure (ERF) do so without receiving any preventive treatment. Late referral of such patients is associated with increased morbidity and mortality, and removes the option of pre-emptive kidney transplantation (Khan *et al.*, 2005). Most patients reaching ERF have progressed through earlier stages of chronic kidney disease (CKD). However, most patients with early CKD do not progress to ERF; the main risk in this group is of premature cardiovascular disease. Both risks can be reduced by treatment of cardiovascular risk factors. The purpose of this article is to enable practitioners in primary and secondary care to recognize the early features of chronic kidney disease, to implement early treatment to prevent its progression and to minimize the cardiovascular risks, and to recognize the minority of patients with progressive kidney damage who will benefit from referral to a nephrologist.

The Department of Health in England has now published a *National Service Framework for Renal Services* (Department of Health, 2004 and 2005); in addition, comprehensive clinical practice guidelines on the identification, management and referral of patients with CKD have recently been published in the UK (Joint Speciality Committee on Renal Disease, 2006; Burden and Tomson, 2005).

Classification of CKD

Table 2.1 outlines the classification scheme adopted by the UK CKD guideline group; this is very similar to classifications used in North America (the Kidney Disease Outcomes Quality Initiative scheme; K/DOQI Clinical Practice Guidelines, 2002) and that proposed by an international working group (Kidney Disease: Improving Global Outcomes (KDIGO)). These schemes have been criticized for giving prominence to estimated glomerular filtration rate (GFR) over other markers of the severity of kidney disease, such as proteinuria and systemic blood pressure. They have also triggered a debate about the extent to which a decline in GFR with age is normal, and what level of GFR should be considered a 'disease' in an elderly person. In addition, the use of the term 'stage' implies that there is an inevitable progression from stage 1 to stage 5, whereas in truth most CKD is non-progressive, and at least some cases of stage 5 CKD occur as a result of irreversible acute renal failure amongst patients whose kidney function may have been completely normal a few days before the precipitating illness. Despite these criticisms, the classification has gained widespread acceptance internationally.

Causes of CKD

To our knowledge the causes of CKD stages 1–3 have not been documented comprehensively at population level with full radiological and biopsy testing; hospital-based series will not be representative. However, information is available on those who start dialysis, the commonest single cause being type 2 diabetes mellitus. Atherosclerotic vascular disease affecting the major renal arteries commonly accompanies CKD in the elderly, but whether this relationship is causal – and whether progression of CKD can be prevented by revascularization – remains uncertain (see Chapter 5). In a large proportion of patients, especially those who present late, it is impossible to give a cause. Amongst both patients with diabetes mellitus and

Table 2.1 Classification scheme adopted by the UK CKD guideline group

	Normalized estimated GFR (mL/min/1.73 m²)	Monitoring	Management	Criteria for referral
Stage 1	>90 + other markers of CKD[a]	Annual BP[b], urine protein, serum creatinine	Advice on CVS risk factors[c] Individualized consideration of aspirin and lipid-lowering drug therapy Antihypertensive therapy	Malignant hypertension Hyperkalaemia (>7 mmol/L) Nephrotic syndrome Isolated proteinuria (protein:creatinine > 100 mg/mmol) Proteinuria and microscopic haematuria (protein:creatinine >45 mg/mmol) Diabetes with increasing proteinuria but without retinopathy Macroscopic haematuria (after negative urological evaluation) Uncontrolled hypertension (e.g. BP >150/90 despite three complementary antihypertensive agents) with a suspicion of underlying kidney disease, including atherosclerotic renal artery stenosis Recurrent pulmonary oedema with normal left ventricular function Fall of estimated GFR of >20% during the first 2 months after initiation of ACEI or ARB treatment
Stage 2[d]	60–89 + other markers of CKD[a]	Annual BP, urine protein, serum creatinine	As above	As above
Stage 3[d]	30–59	6-monthly BP, serum creatinine, Hb, Ca, and PO₄ and urine protein Frequency of monitoring can be reduced to 12-monthly if stable kidney function[e]	As above, plus: Treatment of renal anaemia Renal ultrasonography if patient has symptoms or signs of bladder outflow obstruction[f] Immunization against influenza and pneumococcus Regular review of all prescribed medication, ensuring avoidance of nephrotoxic medications (e.g. NSAIDs), wherever possible Consideration of calcium and vitamin D supplementation: exclude hyperparathyroidism before considering treatment of 'osteoporosis' with antiresorptive drugs	As above, plus: Progressive fall in GFR Microscopic haematuria (after negative urological evaluation if >50 years old) Proteinuria (urine protein:creatinine ratio >45 mg/mmol) Anaemia (after exclusion of bleeding, haematinic deficiency, haemolysis) Persistently abnormal serum potassium, calcium, or phosphate, confirmed on an uncuffed sample Suspected underlying systemic illness, e.g. SLE, vasculitis, myeloma Uncontrolled hypertension (e.g. BP >150/90 despite three complementary antihypertensive agents)
Stage 4[d]	15–29	Three-monthly BP measurement Three-monthly serum creatinine, Hb, Ca, PO₄, HCO₃, PTH	All of the above, plus: Dietary assessment Immunization against hepatitis B Correction of acidosis, if present Treatment of abnormalities of Ca, PO₄, or PTH according to UK CKD guidelines Counselling about all options for treatment Timely provision of vascular or peritoneal access or pre-emptive live donor transplantation, depending on patient's choice of modality	All patients should be discussed formally with a nephrologist and offered the options of RRT or conservative therapy, even if it is not anticipated that RRT will be appropriate, for instance in the presence of another life-threatening illness such as advanced malignancy, or in the presence of advanced dementia.
Stage 5[d]	<15	Most patients will be receiving renal replacement therapy. If not, blood tests as above should be performed at least as frequently as in stage 4.	All of the above	As above. Very few patients should reach stage 5 CKD without previously having been referred, and the management of those that do should be subjected to root cause analysis, i.e. a case by case audit of prior management to identify whether there were missed opportunities for earlier referral.

[a] Other markers of CKD: persistent, laboratory-confirmed microalbuminuria or proteinuria; microscopic or recurrent macroscopic haematuria (after exclusion of other causes, e.g. urological disease); structural abnormalities of the kidneys demonstrated on imaging (e.g. polycystic disease, reflux nephropathy); biopsy-proven glomerulonephritis.

[b] Blood pressure should be measured according to the guidelines of the British Hypertension Society.

[c] CVS risk factors that should be addressed are smoking, obesity, lack of regular aerobic exercise, excessive alcohol intake, and excessive sodium intake.

[d] Acute renal failure must be excluded before a diagnosis of CKD is made.

[e] Stable kidney function: rate of fall of GFR <2 mL/min/1.73 m² over 6 months.

[f] International prostate symptom score >7 or peak urine flow rate <15 mL/min.

ACEI: angiotensin converting enzyme inhibitor; ARB: angiotensin receptor blocker; BP: blood pressure; CKD: chronic kidney disease; CVS: cardiovascular system; GFR: glomerular filtration rate; Hb:

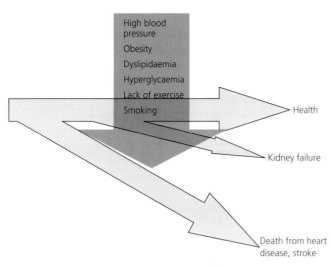

Figure 2.1 The 'competing causes' concept. The same risk factors increase the risk both of fatal cardiovascular disease and of chronic kidney disease. Prevention of cardiovascular deaths may allow more people to live long enough to develop chronic kidney disease.

those with atherosclerosis, reduced death rates, following successful cardiovascular preventive measures, from 'competing causes' such as myocardial infarction may be part of the reason for the apparent 'epidemic' of CKD in affluent countries (Fig. 2.1).

Options for detection of CKD

As discussed in the preceding section, diagnosis of CKD depends on one or more of the following four factors:

- evidence of structural kidney disease;
- haematuria, either known to be of renal origin, or presumed to be after exclusion of other causes;
- proteinuria, including so-called 'microalbuminuria' (see Chapter 1);
- estimated GFR < 60 mL/min/1.73 m² (preferably for two estimations at least three months apart).

In general, renal imaging to detect structural kidney disease will be confined to those with symptoms justifying investigation and those with a family history, for instance of polycystic kidney disease (see Chapter 7) or reflux nephropathy (see Chapter 8). These patients constitute a small minority of patients with CKD.

Dipstick haematuria is known to be present in around 4% of the adult population, of whom at least 50% can be shown to have glomerular disease (most commonly IgA nephropathy or thin basement membrane nephropathy). However, progressive loss of GFR amongst subjects found to have microscopic haematuria of renal origin is extremely rare if GFR is initially normal and proteinuria is absent, and for this reason screening for renal disease using tests for haematuria is not recommended (see Chapter 1).

Any degree of proteinuria, including microalbuminuria, is associated with an increased risk of cardiovascular disease and, at least for patients with diabetes mellitus, with an increased risk of progressive kidney disease. Which test to use for detection of proteinuria depends on the balance between cost and utility. For patients with diabetes mellitus, the observation that angiotensin converting

enzyme inhibitors (ACEIs) and/or angiotensin receptor blockers (ARBs) can reduce and even reverse microalbuminuria, and that this translates into prevention of progressive CKD, justifies laboratory testing – usually using albumin:creatinine ratios on early morning urine samples. Microalbuminuria can also frequently be detected amongst non-diabetic members of the general population, is associated with hypertension and atherosclerosis, and can similarly be reversed by ACEIs or ARBs. However, there is as yet no hard evidence that selective treatment of non-diabetic microalbuminuric patients with these drugs results in long-term benefit. Amongst patients with CKD, more marked proteinuria (e.g. > 1 gram/day or PCR of > 100) is strongly predictive of progressive loss of GFR, and in this situation there is clear evidence that treatment with ACEI or ARBs reduces the risk of progression.

Use of prediction formulae to estimate GFR has revolutionized the approach to detection and treatment of CKD in the community over the last few years. The UK guidelines recommend the use of the 4-variable 'MDRD' formula. This formula has the advantage that, unlike some methods, knowledge of the patient's weight is not required, as the estimate it gives is 'normalized' to body surface area, as is the convention for isotopic measurements of GFR. From April 2006, most UK laboratories have reported an estimate of GFR using this formula every time that they report a serum creatinine concentration. This strategy alone will greatly increase the recognition of CKD in the community, necessitating a coherent strategy for management of all the patients in whom CKD is newly recognized. The strategy has also re-focused attention on marked variations between laboratories in the calibration of creatinine assays (see Chapter 1).

Epidemiology of CKD

Two large population-based studies of the prevalence of CKD are available. Data from the National Health and Nutrition Survey in the USA gave an estimate of 11%, based on estimated GFR and albumin excretion (Table 2.1). A survey in Australia also included haematuria as a diagnostic criterion; here the estimated prevalence of CKD was 16%. There are no equivalent population-based epidemiological studies from the UK, but studies based on laboratory testing, which inevitably underestimate prevalence, are consistent with these figures. These studies have changed our perception of CKD, which was previously thought to be relatively rare. Patients with CKD are predominantly elderly. CKD is less common amongst people of white European descent than amongst those from ethnic minority populations; in the UK, it is three to four times more common amongst the Afro-Caribbean and South Asian population, in whom hypertension and diabetes mellitus, respectively, are largely responsible for the difference.

The risk of premature death, particularly from cardiovascular disease, is greatly increased amongst people with CKD. This is partly because classical cardiovascular risk factors (hypertension, sedentary lifestyle, obesity, cigarette smoking, dyslipidaemia) also promote the development and progression of CKD. Whether CKD itself is an independent risk factor that accelerates the progression of atherosclerosis, via the operation of novel CKD-specific risk factors, is uncertain. The association between CKD and cardiovascular disease may be due to different mechanisms in people with albuminuria but normal GFR and in those with reduced GFR with or without albuminuria. Both groups have been excluded from many of the randomized controlled trials on which recommendations for lipid-lowering therapy are based, so it remains uncertain whether CKD should be an indication for such therapy if it would otherwise not be indicated according to the Joint British Societies guidelines (see www.bhsoc.org/Other_Guidelines.stm).

Selective screening for CKD

Certain groups are at significantly increased risk of CKD. Because the early stages of CKD are asymptomatic, and early intervention can prevent progression of CKD and also reduce the risk of cardiovascular disease, selective screening for markers of CKD is recommended (Joint Speciality Committee on Renal Disease, 2006; Burden and Tomson, 2005).

Management and referral of CKD

Most patients with CKD have co-existing conditions, particularly diabetes mellitus and hypertension; only a small minority progress to stage 5, but detection and timely referral of these is extremely important. Specialist input also adds value in some other groups; criteria for referral are summarized in Table 2.1. For the majority of patients with CKD, specialist referral is neither practicable nor necessary, and could even contribute to disease-based fragmentation of care as well as diverting resources away from those who would benefit from additional specialist input. These patients need integrated, community-based chronic disease management, with a well-defined system for ensuring long-term follow-up. Electronic decision support to guide therapy at each stage of CKD is being developed, based on the UK guidelines (see http://www.renal.org/ckd).

Further reading

Burden R, Tomson C. (2005) Identification, management, and referral of adults with chronic kidney disease: concise guidelines. *Clinical Medicine*; **5**: 635–42.

Department of Health (2004) *The National Service Framework for Renal Services. Part One: Dialysis and Transplantation*, pp. 1–50. Department of Health, London.

Department of Health (2005) *National Service Framework for Renal Services. Part Two: Chronic Kidney Disease, Acute Renal Failure, and End of Life Care*, pp. 1–30. Department of Health, London.

Joint Specialty Committee on Renal Disease of the Royal College of Physicians of London and the Renal Association (2006) *Chronic Kidney Disease in Adults: UK Guidelines for Identification, Management, and Referral*. Royal College of Physicians of London, London.

Kidney Disease Outcome Quality Initiative (2002) K/DOQI clinical practice guidelines for chronic kidney disease: evaluation, classification, and stratification. *American Journal of Kidney Disorders*; **390** (2, Suppl 2): S1–S246.

Khan SS, Xue JL, Kazmi WH *et al.* (2005) Does predialysis nephrology care influence patient survival after initiation of dialysis? *Kidney International*; **67**(3): 1038–46.

CHAPTER 3

Chronic Kidney Disease – Prevention of Progression and of Cardiovascular Complications

Mohsen El Kossi, Aminu Kasarawa Bello, Rizwan Hamer, A Meguid El Nahas

OVERVIEW

- In the UK, around 100 patients per million population/year are started on renal replacement therapy (RRT). Provision of RRT will consume about 2% of the NHS budget in the next decade.

- Individuals with stages 1 to 4 are likely to exceed by greater than 50-fold those reaching ERF (stage 5).

- It is estimated that 11% of the adult American population may have CKD.

- The trend of CKD risk factors/markers (which include diabetes, hypertension, obesity, smoking and aging population) is growing, which will possibly result in a consequent increase in CKD rates.

- The majority of CKD sufferers succumb to cardiovascular disease.

- Diabetic kidney disease, glomerular diseases, polycystic kidney disease are associated with a faster GFR decline than hypertensive and tubulointerstitial kidney diseases.

- The control of systemic hypertension is the most effective intervention to slow the progression of CKD. Current guidelines recommend a reduction in BP to below 130/80 mmHg in patients with CKD although lower BP targets (< 125/75 mmHg) have been advocated for patients with heavy proteinuria and those with diabetic nephropathy.

- Protein/albumin is thought to have a direct nephrotoxic effect. Angiotensin converting enzyme inhibitors and angiotensin receptor blockers probably have a therapeutic advantage as they are effective at reducing both hypertension and proteinuria.

- In diabetic patients, poor glycaemic control appears to contribute to a faster rate of decline of diabetic nephropathy.

- Cost both in quality of life and financially, plus cost of co-morbidities associated with CKD, makes it imperative that renal disease is detected early and managed meticulously to prevent its progression.

- Complications of CKD include:
  - cardiovascular disease;
  - malnutrition;
  - anaemia;
  - hypertension;
  - hyperparathyroidism and consequent renal osteodystrophy.

Background

An increasing number of patients are being treated worldwide for chronic kidney disease (CKD). Globally, it has been suggested that as many as 100 million individuals may be affected. The natural course of CKD extends from being susceptible to the disease, exposed to the risk factors and to development of CKD and progression to established renal failure (ERF) needing renal replacement therapy (RRT) or leading to death. A better understanding of the epidemiology, risk factors and natural history of CKD is likely to lead to better prevention and management of this rising healthcare threat.

CKD: epidemiolology

Provision of care for patients who require dialysis or transplantation is a major and growing healthcare problem in both developed and emerging nations in terms of cost, premature mortality and economic impact. It is estimated that over 1.5 million patients with ERF worldwide are currently on RRT with the number due to exceed 2 million by 2010, at a global cost of around a trillion dollars. Ninety percent of all treated ERF patients reside in the West as the prohibitive cost precludes RRT in most developing nations. In the USA, it is estimated that RRT will cost around $29 billion by 2010. Currently, in the UK around 100 patients per million population (pmp)/year are started on RRT. Provision of RRT may consume about 2% of the NHS cost in the next decade.

There are geographical differences in the causes and prevalence of ERF (Table 3.1). The reasons for these observed discrepancies in the incidence and prevalence of ERF are multi-factorial, ranging from racial and socio-economic factors as well as health services development and provision. Information from developing countries in Asia, Africa and South America is scarce due to lack of renal registries and database and the fact that their economies cannot sustain the growing burden of ERF. In fact, 110 of 222 world countries are unable to provide RRT leaving more than 600 million individuals without treatment for ERF. Consequently, around 1 million individuals die every year from untreated ERF.

Of major concern is the fact that the number of patients with ERF is a small proportion of the entire burden of CKD, as individuals with earlier stages (1 to 4) are likely to exceed by greater than 50-fold those reaching ERF (stage 5). In the USA, the third National Health and Nutrition Examination Survey (NHANES III) has estimated that 11% (19 millions) of the adult American population may have CKD. Of these, only 300 000 have reached CKD stage 5 (ERF). The burden of CKD may also be high in countries such as the UK, Netherlands, Australia and in some developing countries

Table 3.1 Incidence and prevalence of established renal failure (ERF) in different countries

Country	Incidence (pmp/year)	Prevalence (pmp/year)
UK	104	632
Europe (average)	135	700
Australia:		
General population	125	685
Aboriginal/Torres Strait Islanders	379	1987
New Zealand:		
General population	140	715
Aboriginal	231	1139
USA:		
All	338	1500
Black	989	4700
White	256	1096
China		
National average	15	33
Shanghai	102	180
Russia	15	79

Most data are for the period between 2001 and 2005.

such as India, and Singapore (Table 3.2). However, many of those with signs of CKD have underlying hypertension and/or diabetes mellitus often previously unrecognized or poorly controlled.

CKD: future burden and projection forecast

There are few estimates on the future burden of CKD. Globalization and risk transition phenomena have evolved with a growing trend in CKD risk factors/markers such as diabetes, hypertension, obesity, and smoking, and therefore possible consequent increase in CKD rates. For example, the current global diabetes population of 154 million is expected to double in the next two decades. The prevalence of hypertension is projected to increase by 60% in the next two decades, affecting one third of the world adult population. One fifth of the world population (1.6 billion) is overweight or obese and 1.3 billion smoke cigarettes. Changes in lifestyle and population demographics, such as aging, may also impact on the increasing trend of CKD in the coming decades.

CKD risk factors

The susceptibility, initiation and progression of CKD are all associated with risk markers/factors (Table 3.3). The former refers to observed associations whilst the latter refers to causal ones. Some of the risk markers/factors are implicated in both susceptibility and progression; many are also associated with increased cardiovascular (CVD) risk. Susceptibility to CKD is higher among certain families and races. This highlights the possibility of genetic predisposition to CKD. In the USA, racial differences in the prevalence of CKD and ERF may reflect the high prevalence of hypertension- and diabetes-related CKD amongst Native and African-Americans. In the UK, Afro-Caribbeans and Indo-Asians are at increased risk of CKD. One elegant hypothesis links low birth weight amongst ethnic minorities to consequent fetal renal underdevelopment and a reduced number of hypertrophied nephrons (oligomeganephronia). These birth defects may, in adult life, contribute to the pathogenesis of hypertension and CKD. Male gender and older age groups are also more susceptible to the development of CKD. Amongst the known risk factors for the initiation of CKD are hypertension, diabetes, hyperlipidaemia, obesity and smoking. In

Table 3.2 Prevalence of chronick kidney disease (CKD) markers in some community-based studies

Country	N	Population category	CKD prevalence (%)	Proteinuria/albuminuria (%)	GFR <60mL/min (%)	ERF (%)
UK:						
KEAPS	425	At-risk	–	7.1	–	–
EPIC-Norfolk	23964	General	–	12	–	–
USA:						
NHANES III	15625	General	11	6.3	4.3	0.20
KEEP	25000	At-risk	>40	27	16	0.40
Zuni Indians	1483	At-risk	37.5	20	–	2
Netherlands:						
PREVEND	40856	General	–	7.2	–	–
Australia:						
AUSDIAB	11247	General	16	2.4	11.2	–
Tiwi Aborigines	237	At-risk	56	44	12	–
Singapore: NKF Study	450000	General		0.8		

KEAPS: Kidney Early Evaluation Program in Sheffield (unpublished data). EPIC-Norfolk: Epic-Norfolk Prospective Population Study. NHANES III: Third National Health and Nutrition Examination Survey. KEEP: Kidney Early Evaluation Program. Ausdiab: the Australian Diabetes, Obesity and Lifestyle study. PREVEND: Prevention of Renal and Vascular End Stage Disease Study. NKF: the National Kidney Foundation Singapore. Tiwi: Australian Aboriginal Community Study. Zuni: Zuni Pueblo Community Study.
ERF: established renal failure; GFR: glomerular filtration rate.

developing countries, the profile of risk factors for initiation of CKD may also reflect the impact of communicable disease such as HIV, hepatitis C, malaria, schistosomiasis as well as tuberculosis.

CKD: natural history and progression

The rate of progression and GFR decline in CKD is very variable. In the majority of patients there is little or no progression, with the majority of CKD sufferers succumbing to cardiovascular disease. Some types of kidney diseases, however, progress significantly. Diabetic kidney disease, glomerular diseases and polycystic kidney disease are associated with a faster GFR decline than hypertensive and tubulointerstitial kidney diseases. Irrespective of the original kidney disease, there are other modifiable and non-modifiable risk factors which influence the rate of CKD progression. African-American race (USA), diabetic Asians (UK), lower baseline level of kidney function, male gender, and older age are among the non-modifiable risk factors associated with a faster GFR decline. Hypertension is the single most important risk factors associated with accelerated decline in kidney function in CKD patients. The control of systemic hypertension is the most effective intervention to slow the progression of CKD. Current guidelines recommend a reduction in blood pressure to levels below 130/80 mmHg in patients with CKD. Furthermore, lower blood pressure targets < 125/75 mmHg, have been advocated for patients with heavy proteinuria > 1 g/24 h, and those suffering from diabetic nephropathy. Heavy proteinuria is also associated with a faster rate of decline attributed by some to a direct nephrotoxic effect of protein/albumin on renal tubules. With that in mind, it is imperative that the control of hypertension is coupled with a reduction in proteinuria to levels less than 1 g/24 h.

Angiotensin converting enzyme inhibitors and angiotensin receptor blockers may have a therapeutic advantage as they are effective at reducing both hypertension and proteinuria. In diabetic patients, poor glycaemic control appears to contribute to a faster rate of decline of diabetic nephropathy. Target glycosylated haemoglobin levels around < 7% are recommended. Dyslipidaemia and smoking are also among the modifiable risk factors associated with a progressive CKD and have to be addressed (Tables 3.3 and 3.4).

Many, if not all, of the risk factors/markers associated with progressive CKD have also been implicated in CVD. Furthermore, albuminuria has recently been identified as a strong marker for cardiovascular disease morbidity and mortality. The PREVEND study showed increased cardiovascular mortality in the general population with

Table 3.3 Risk markers/factors for chronic kidney disease

Non-modifiable	Modifiable
Old age (S)	Systemic hypertension (I, P)
Male sex (S)	Diabetes mellitus (I, P)
Race/ethnicity (S)	Proteinuria (P)
Genetic predisposition (S)	Dyslipidaemia (I, P)
Family history (S)	Smoking (I, P)
Low birth weight (S)	Obesity (I, P)
	Alcohol consumption (I, P)
	Low socio-economic status (S)
	Infections/infestations (I)
	Drugs and herbs/analgesic abuse (I)
	Autoimmune diseases/obstructive uropathy/ stones (I)

S: Susceptibility factor, I: Initiation factor, P: Progression factor.

Table 3.4 Complications of chronic kidney disease (CKD) and interventions to prevent them

Complications of CKD (Intervention targets)	Interventions
Cardiovascular disease (Minimize left ventricular hypertrophy Prevent congestive heart failure)	Control hypertension (< 130/80 mmHg; < 125/75 mmHg if proteinuria > 1 g/day) ACEI/ARB as indicated – preferential if proteinuria > 1 g/day Control dyslipidaemia/statins – secondary prevention of existing CV disease : total cholesterol < 4 mmol/L and LDL-cholesterol < 2.0 mmol/L Correct anaemia (see below) Control hyperparathyroidism (see below) Cessation of smoking
Anaemia (see Appendix 2) (Hb: 10.5–12.5 g/dL. Avoid drop of Hb below 10 g/dL)	Correct haematinic deficiencies Supplement with (oral/parenteral) iron in CKD 4–5 Treat with erythropoietin in CKD 4–5
Renal osteodystrophy (Serum calcium: > 2.2 mmol/L; serum phosphorus: < 1.8 mmol/L; PTH: normal– twice normal level)	Reduce phosphate intake: ~ 800 mg/day Consider phosphate binders Calcium and vitamin D supplementation
Malnutrition	Adequate protein/calories supplementation Correct metabolic acidosis Timely initiation of RRT (GFR ~ 10 mL/min) (see Chapter 10)

ACEI: angiotension converting enzyme inhibitor; ARB: angiotensin receptor blocker; GFR: glomerular filtration rate; HB: haemoglobin; PTH: Parathyroid hormone; RRT: renal replacement therapy.

increased urine albumin excretion rate. This has also been observed in studies of patients with coronary artery disease and hypertension, where albuminuria was noted to be a stronger predictor of cardiovascular morbidity than some of the better-known CVD markers such as hypertension or hyperlipidaemia. Therefore population screening for albuminuria may have the advantage of early detection of those at risk of both CKD and CVD. It is most likely that cost-effective screening programmess will focus on the at-risk population including hypertensive, diabetic and obese individuals. In addition, screening of the elderly for proteinuria is more cost-effective than those under the age of 60 in view of the higher prevalence of CKD in the elderly.

Detailed recommendations for the screening and detection of early CKD are made in Chapter 2.

Concerted effort is warranted to detect and prevent the progression of CKD. This would have major healthcare impacts as well as considerable socio-economic consequences. Such an approach is the sole approach applicable to many developing countries where CKD and its progression to ERF equates to a death sentence (see Chapter 12).

Complications of CKD

The interventions discussed above are primarily aimed to slow the progression of CKD. It is important to appreciate that the outcome and prognosis of patients with ERF is often determined by associated uraemic complications, including CVD and malnutrition at the initiation of RRT. Cardiovascular complications include coronary artery disease, heart failure and left ventricular hypertrophy; if these are present at the initiation of RRT this confers a poor long-term prognosis. In order to minimize CKD-associated CVD, anaemia, hypertension and hyperparathyroidism, including the calcium/phosphate balance, need to be corrected (Table 3.4). In order to minimize malnutrition, attention needs to be paid to the optimization of dietary protein and caloric intake. Metabolic acidosis has a significant catabolic effect and should be corrected. Other complications of CKD also need to be addressed, including the early management of renal osteodystrophy. The control of hyperphosphataemia and the reduction of raised calcium phosphate product may also have an impact on the progression of CVD-associated morbidity and mortality. Finally, timely referral for evaluation of the best way to manage progressive renal functional decline (e.g. pre-emptive renal transplantation (see Chapter 11), the initiation of planned RRT (see Chapter 10) or conservative therapy (see Chapter 9) is essential in patients close to or at stage 5 CKD). Most guidelines recommend starting RRT at a GFR around $10 \, mL/min/1.73 \, m^2$.

In conclusion, CKD is a growing healthcare problem that is preventable, detectable and manageable with careful strategic planning and optimal and timely interventions.

Further reading

Coresh J, Astor BC, Greene T, Eknoyan G, Levey AS. (2003) Prevalence of chronic kidney disease and decreased kidney function in the adult US population: Third National Health and Nutrition Examination Survey. *American Journal of Kidney Disease*; **41**: 1–12.

De Vecchi AF, Dratwa M, Wiedmann ME. (1999) Healthcare systems and end-stage renal disease. An international review: Costs and reimbursement of ESRD therapies. *New England Journal of Medicine*; **14**: 31–41.

El Nahas AM, Bello AK. (2005) Chronic kidney disease: the global challenge. *Lancet*; **365**: 331–40.

Kidney Disease Outcome Quality Initiative (2002) K/DOQI clinical practice guidelines for chronic kidney disease: evaluation, classification, and stratification. *American Journal of Kidney Disease*; **39** (2, Suppl. 2): S1–246.

Lysaght, MJ. (2002) Maintenance dialysis population dynamics: Current trends and long-term implications. *Journal of the American Society of Nephrology*; **13**: 37–40.

UK Renal Registry (2004) *The Seventh Annual Report* [WWW document]. URL http://www.renalreg.com [Accessed on 21 December 2005].

CHAPTER 4

Adult Nephrotic Syndrome

Richard Hull, Sean Gallagher, David Goldsmith

OVERVIEW

- Nephrotic syndrome is a common condition in kidney specialist practice with significant complications. It is caused by a wide range of primary (idiopathic) and secondary glomerular diseases.
- Patients can present in various clinical settings, with not insignificant numbers undergoing community-based treatment with care shared between specialists and primary care.
- All patients need referral to a nephrologist for further investigation with a renal biopsy.
- Initial management should be focused at investigating its cause, identifying complications and managing the presenting symptoms of the disease.
- No conclusive evidence currently exists for the best treatment strategies for most primary glomerular diseases.

Nephrotic syndrome

The nephrotic syndrome (NS) is one of the best-known presentations of adult or paediatric kidney disease (Orth *et al.*, 1998). It describes the association of heavy *proteinuria* with *peripheral oedema, hypoalbuminaemia* and *hyperlipidaemia* (Box 4.1a,b). NS has multiple causes, significant complications and it requires referral to a nephrologist for further investigation and management. Patients can present *de novo* in various clinical settings, with not insignificant numbers of patients undergoing community-based treatment, with management shared between specialists and primary care (the paradigm for much of renal medicine in the twenty-first century).

Though NS is a common condition in nephrological practice and should feature in the differential diagnosis of any oedematous patient, there can be uncertainty about how best to manage it. In part this is due to a lack of randomized controlled trials, and the presence of only a handful of Cochrane systematic reviews.

Box 4.1a Diagnostic criteria for nephrotic syndrome

- Greater than 3–3.5 g/24hr proteinuria or spot urine protein creatinine ratio (PCR) of > 300–350 mg/mmol
- Serum albumin < 25 g/L
- Clinical evidence of peripheral oedema
- Can also be associated with hyperlipidaemia (raised total cholesterol) and lipiduria

Box 4.1b Definition and classification of proteinuria (see Chapter 1)

- Transient increased proteinuria can be seen in fever, post-exercise, post-seizure, in severe acute illnesses.
- Persistent proteinuria of > 150 mg/day (PCR ~ 10-20 mg/mmol) implies renal or systemic disease.
- Dipsticks predominantly detect urinary albumin (and are positive if excretion is > 300 mg/day).

This chapter provides an update on the management of NS in adults. We review relevant investigation and therapeutic strategies for the general condition of NS, and for some of the primary glomerular causes (but we deliberately avoid highly-specialized or recherché conditions). In particular, our approach emphasizes the clinical challenges faced by doctors without specialized renal experience when presented with a patient with suspected NS.

It is helpful to have in mind when considering renal oedema, salt and water retention, and the action of diuretics an understanding of renal anatomy, and renal physiology, at the level described in Figure 4.1.

Conditions causing nephrotic syndrome

NS is caused by a wide range of conditions that can be classified as primary (idiopathic) glomerular (Table 4.1) or secondary diseases (Box 4.2).

Primary (idiopathic) glomerular disease

Primary glomerular diseases account for the majority of cases of NS. Thirty years ago, idiopathic membranous nephropathy (see Appendix 1) was the most common primary cause. The incidence of the other glomerular pathologies, particularly focal segmental glomerulosclerosis (FSGS) (see Appendix 1), has increased. There are marked racial associations with different underlying primary glomerular diseases – membranous nephropathy is the most frequent cause of NS in Caucasians whilst FSGS is the most common amongst black patients, with a frequency of 50-57% of cases (Haas *et al.*, 1997; Korbet *et al.*, 1996).

Secondary glomerular disease

A wide range of diseases and drugs can cause NS. Secondary causes can often give a similar or identical histological lesion to a primary

Table 4.1 Primary glomerular diseases causing the nephrotic syndrome

Disease	Frequency of disease (%)		
	Classic data		Modern data
	<60yr	>60yr	
Focal segmental glomerulosclerosis	15	2	35
Membranous	40	39	33
Minimal change	20	20	15
Membranoproliferative, e.g. IgA	7	0	14
Other diseases	18	39	3

(Data adapted from Haas *et al.*, 1997 and Orth & Ritx, 1998)

Box 4.2 **Secondary causes of nephrotic syndrome**

- **Diabetes mellitus**
- **Neoplasia**
- **Drugs**
  - gold
  - antimicrobials
  - NSAIDs
  - penicillamine
  - captopril
  - tamoxifen
  - lithium
- **Infections**
  - HIV
  - hepatitis B and C
  - mycoplasma
  - syphilis
  - malaria
  - schistosomiasis
  - filariasis
  - toxoplasmosis
- **Systemic lupus erythematosus (SLE)**
- **Amyloid**
- **Miscellaneous**

---

disease but have an identifiable underlying pathological process. Diabetic nephropathy is, and will remain, the commonest cause. Amyloid is also an important cause of NS; in one series AL amyloid nephropathy accounted for 10% of cases (Haas *et al.*, 1997).

The patho-physiological reasons for the nephrotic syndrome

The size-selective and charge-selective filtration barrier of the glomerulus prevents the passage of proteins across it. There are three layers: the fenestrated endothelium, the glomerular basement membrane and podocytes with the slit diaphragm between their foot processes (Figs 4.2 and 4.3). NS develops from protein leakage caused by injuries to this barrier. These alter its charge and size selectivity through effects on podocytes by immune and non-immune

mechanisms, and to the expression of vital adhesion molecules such as nephrin.

Explanations for oedema in NS

The underlying process behind sodium retention and oedema formation is complex, controversial, and not fully resolved. The classic 'underfill' hypothesis proposes that low plasma oncotic pressure resulting from proteinuria and hypoalbuminaemia leads to intravascular volume depletion. The physiological response, via the renin-angiotensin-aldosterone and sympathetic nervous systems, causes sodium retention and thus oedema. There are many clinical and experimental studies that tried to validate this theory; a detailed exposition is beyond the scope of this review (Deschênes *et al.*, 2003; Koomans, 2003). The alternative 'overfill' theory proposes that the processes causing sodium retention are intrarenal, primarily in the collecting duct of the nephron (Ichikawa *et al.*, 1983). There are still

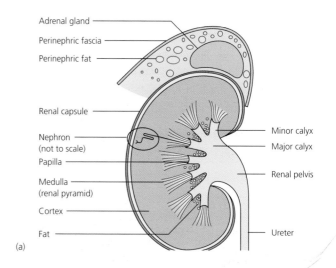

(a)

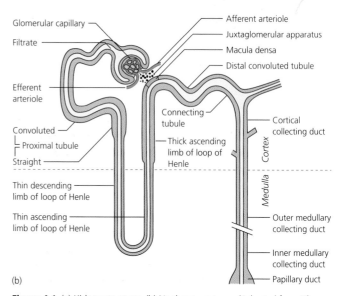

(b)

Figure 4.1 (a) Kidney structure. (b) Nephron anatomy. (Adapted from *The Renal System at a Glance*, with permission of Blackwell Publishing Ltd.)

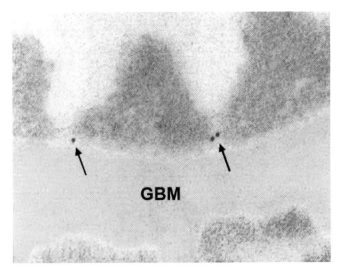

Figure 4.2 Glomerular slit diaphragm. (Reproduced with permission from Institute of Biotechnology, Helsinki.)

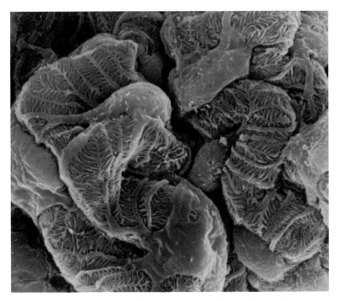

Figure 4.3 Electron micrograph of podocyte cells. (Reproduced with permission from Steve Gschmeissner/Science Photo Library.)

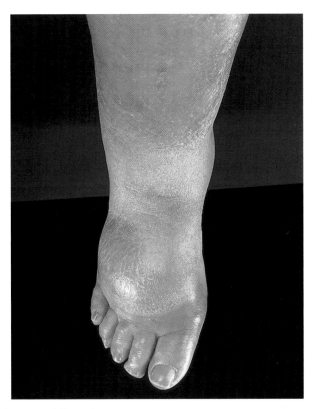

Figure 4.4 Pitting oedema.

the body result in many of the complications seen. It is important for the clinician to be aware of their potential and actively prevent their occurrence.

Risk of thromboembolism

NS results in a hypercoagulable state with an increased risk of thromboembolic events. Embolism affect up to 10% of adults in clinical series of NS (Nolasco *et al.*, 1986). Multiple abnormalities in the coagulation system occur including increased plasma levels of pro-coagulant factors, reduced plasma levels of anti-coagulant factors, abnormal platelet function, altered endothelial function and decreased fibrinolytic activity. Intravascular volume depletion, an increase in

unanswered questions and indeed one rather more pragmatic view is that sodium retention leading to oedema formation (Fig. 4.4) is likely to result from a spectrum of pathogenic mechanisms; some 'underfill' and some 'overfill' (Hamm and Batuman, 2003).

Complications of nephrotic syndrome

The nephrotic syndrome has systemic consequences (Box 4.3). Not infrequently, the first manifestation of NS can be a complication, such as deep venous thrombosis, breathlessness or infection. There is overproduction of proteins in the liver (as part of the hepatic response to hypoalbuminaemia) and loss of low molecular weight proteins in the urine. Significant changes in the protein environment of

Box 4.3 **Complications of nephrotic syndrome**

- Thromboembolism:
  - DVT +/− pulmonary embolism;
  - renal vein;
  - arterial (rare).
- Infection:
  - cellulitis;
  - bacterial peritonitis (rare);
  - bacterial infections, e.g. pneumonia;
  - viral infections in the immunocompromised.
- Hyperlipidaemia;
- Malnutrition;
- Acute renal failure.

haematocrit from diuretics, and immobilization, are significant contributory factors.

The most common sites of thrombosis in adults are the deep veins of the lower limb. This is often asymptomatic. Renal vein thrombosis (RVT) is a well recognized though uncommon complication of NS and is said to be more common when NS is caused by membranous nephropathy or amyloidosis. Pulmonary embolism is also a potential consequence. Arterial thrombosis, affecting mesenteric, axillary, femoral, ophthalmic, renal, pulmonary and coronary arteries has also been (much more rarely) reported.

Infection

Infection can occur in up to 20% of adult patients with NS and is a significant cause of morbidity and, occasionally, mortality. Patients have an increased susceptibility to infection from low serum IgG concentrations, reduced complement activity and depression of T cell function (Ogi *et al.*, 1994).

A variety of infectious complications, particularly bacterial, can occur. Cellulitis is common, especially in severely oedematous limbs, due to skin splits or punctures. Spontaneous bacterial peritonitis is a serious but rare infection in adults. It can present insidiously with mild abdominal colicky pain or as fulminant sepsis. *Streptococcus pneumoniae* and gram-negative organisms are the most frequent causative bacteria. Viral infections have been linked to relapses in minimal change nephrotic syndrome. Infections are a risk in patients receiving immunosuppressive treatment for NS.

Acute renal failure

This is a rare complication of NS. It can happen as a consequence of excessive diuresis, interstitial nephritis related to diuretic or NSAID use, sepsis and renal vein thrombosis. It can happen spontaneously, usually at presentation and occurs more often in the elderly. Patients can require dialysis and can take weeks to months to recover (Crew *et al.*, 2004).

Assessing the patient presenting with nephrotic syndrome

The key aims are to assess the current clinical state of the patient ensuring no complications are present, and to begin to formulate whether there is a primary or secondary cause underlying the syndrome. The vast majority of patients will require referral to a nephrologist for further management including (in adults) a renal biopsy. Patients can present with complications of the syndrome with the actual diagnosis being made later (e.g. DVT).

History

A thorough and careful history is important in elucidating the cause of NS. Patients can notice breathlessness, leg and facial swelling, and, more rarely, frothy urine (protein acting like a detergent in the urine (Fig. 4.5). Particular note should be made of any features suggestive of systemic disease, e.g. systemic lupus erythematosus, drug history (especially any recent or new medications, be they prescribed or 'over the counter') as well as any acute or chronic infections. It is important to remember the links with malignancy particularly of the lungs and large bowel. A history of chronic inflammation may point towards a diagnosis of secondary amyloid. A family history is also important, as there are a number of congenital causes of nephrotic syndrome.

Clinical signs

Patients usually present with increasing peripheral oedema (Fig. 4.4). Up to four litres of fluid can remain clinically undetectable. Oedema is often first noticed peri-orbitally and it can become very severe with lower leg and genital oedema as well as ascites, pleural and pericardial effusions. It is important to mention to the non-specialist that neither raised BP, nor elevated jugular venous pressure/pulmonary oedema, are 'cardinal' features of NS. If these are present, it is more likely that one is dealing with (acute) nephritic syndrome (e.g. secondary to acute glomerulonephritis), or there is significant cardiac or renal failure. The blood pressure in NS can be low, normal or raised – this depends on many factors including previous history of raised BP, underlying cause of NS, renal function, extracellular fluid volume status and cardiac function.

Features of the underlying disorder may be evident, such as the butterfly facial rash of SLE or the neuropathy and retinopathy associated with diabetes mellitus.

Hyperlipidaemia is one of the classic accompaniments to the condition and eruptive xanthomas can appear. The nails can show white bands due to persistent hypoalbuminaemia (Fig. 4.6).

Investigations

Initial investigations (Box 4.4) help establish the current clinical status and pin down the underlying cause of the NS. Key steps include assessment of the renal function through measurement of serum

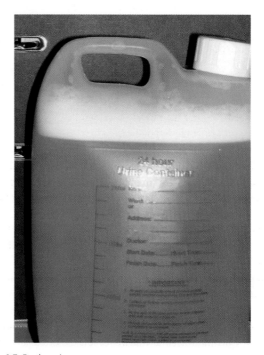

Figure 4.5 Frothy urine.

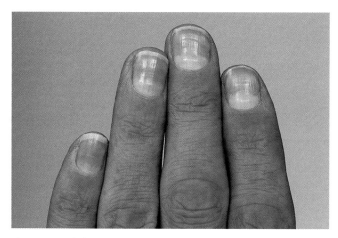

Figure 4.6 Nail changes.

urea and creatinine and an eGFR. The urine should be assessed for the presence of haematuria (suggesting glomerulonephritis) and proteinuria (3 plus protein indicates nephrotic range). It is important to measure the amount of protein being excreted. A spot urine sample for a protein:creatinine ratio (PCR) is almost as accurate, less prone to error, and gives quicker results than a 24 h urine collection (Gaspari *et al.*, 2006). Nephrotic-range proteinuria is defined as a PCR greater than 300–350 mg/mmol. A renal ultrasound, giving an assessment of renal size and morphology should be performed early, and should be done urgently if there is suspicion of renal vein thrombosis.

General treatment measures for nephrotic syndrome

Oedema

The underlying cause of the oedema is sodium retention. The aim of therapy is to create a negative sodium balance. Dietary sodium limitation (< 100 mmol/day), fluid restriction and diuretics may all be needed. Oedema should be reversed by engineering a steady diuresis to cause a weight loss of around 0.5–1 kg/day (and so daily weight is an important metric). More zealous diuresis can precipitate acute renal failure from volume depletion, electrolyte disturbances (hyponatraemia, hypokalaemia) and thrombo-embolism due to haemoconcentration.

Loop diuretics such as furosemide or bumetamide are commonly used. Starting doses should be in the 'conventional' range (e.g. 40–80 mg of furosemide orally). Oedema of the gut wall can affect the absorption of diuretics; refractory cases respond best to larger doses of intravenous loop diuretics. Intravenous boluses or preferably infusions (of much higher doses) of loop diuretics are commonly used; there can be severe side-effects from large (intravenous) doses of loop diuretics (e.g. electrolyte derangement, deafness, or photo-sensitive skin blistering), so care must be taken.

To try to improve on poor responses found with loop diuretics, thiazide diuretics or potassium-sparing diuretics are often added to treatment regimens. A typical additional agent is metolazone (2.5– 5 mg daily). These agents inhibit downstream sodium reabsorp-

Box 4.4 Investigations in the nephrotic patient

Haematology
- full blood count;
- coagulation screen;
- ESR.

Chemistry
- urea and electrolytes including eGFR;
- LFT including albumin;
- bone profile;
- lipid profile;
- glucose;
- CRP;
- spot urine for protein:creatinine ratio (preferably early morning).

Microbiology
- Hepatitis B and C and HIV serology (after appropriate consenting);
- MSU;
- blood cultures if there is fever (> 38 °C).

Immunology
- anti-nuclear antibody (ANA);
- anti-double-stranded DNA antibody (dsDNA);
- complement levels (C3 and C4);
- serum immunoglobulins and electrophoresis;
- urine for Bence Jones Protein.

Radiology
- renal ultrasound;
- CXR
- other imaging (dependent on clinical signs and suspicion of malignancy).

tion and thus work in synergy with loop diuretics which induce a more proximal natriuresis (Fig. 4.7). This loop diuretic–thiazide combination can be tremendously effective, and so requires careful oversight usually in hospital, with daily weight, BP and electrolyte monitoring.

Although intravenous (salt-poor) albumin infusion has often been used to improve or initiate diuresis (working, it is surmised, by increasing the delivery of the diuretic to its site of action through increasing the amount of plasma-bound drug, and by expanding plasma volume), this practice is not supported by evidence from studies. There are potential harmful consequences flowing from the use of intravenous albumin, such as anaphylaxis, hypertension, and pulmonary oedema (Mees, 1996).

Proteinuria

One of the main goals of treatment is the reduction or elimination of proteinuria. Proteinuria is the best independent predictor of progression in all renal disease (Ruggenenti *et al.*, 1998). Strategies to limit protein excretion will also serve to help correct oedema. In some patients this can be achieved by treating the underlying pathology but in the majority of patients the proteinuria needs active control. The general measures used usually achieve proteinuria reduction by also causing a reduction in GFR. A number of older treatments, for example high-dose NSAIDs, have signifi-

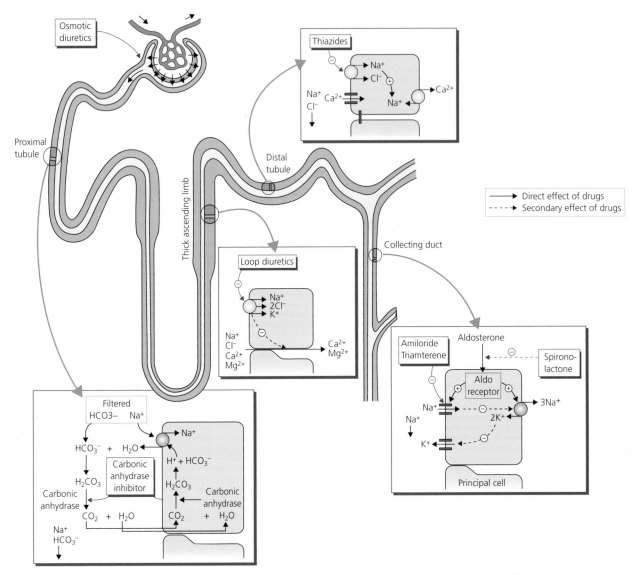

Figure 4.7 Site of action of diuretics in the kidney. (Adapted from *The Renal System at a Glance,* with permission from Blackwell Publishing Ltd.)

cant side-effects and are rarely used now. Low protein diets have not shown consistent results in reducing proteinuria, and are not recommended.

Proteinuria is linked to blood pressure – for heavily nephrotic patients a BP of < 125/75 mmHg is ideal. Proteinuria is also linked to obesity, so weight loss in chronically heavily proteinuric obese subjects is desirable.

Angiotensin converting enzyme (ACE) inhibitors, either on their own or in conjunction with angiotensin II receptor antagonists, are the mainstay of anti-BP/anti-proteinuric therapy. The dose response curve in this setting is different to their anti-hypertensive effects (which can mean using larger doses) and it can often take some weeks for their full effect to be manifest. Proteinuria reduction can be seen in the absence of any effect on systemic blood pressure; combination therapy reduces proteinuria more effectively than single agents alone (Nakao *et al.*, 2003; Tsouli *et al.*, 2006). Using these agents mandates regular monitoring of plasma electrolytes (also mandatory when large diuretic doses are employed).

It should not be forgotten that indapamide, and non-dihydropyridine calcium-channel blockers such as verapamil and diltiazem, are all anti-proteinuric anti-hypertensives, and these can also usefully be added to ACEI-based regimens.

In extreme cases, where the proteinuria is severe and uncontrollable leading to incapacitating symptoms from, or complications of, NS (e.g. renal dysfunction or malnutrition), it is possible to use nephrectomy or renal arterial embolization. In practice these extreme measures are very rarely needed in adults.

Thromboembolism – prevention and treatment

Any confirmed thrombosis needs systemic anticoagulation with heparin and then warfarin. Higher doses than normal of heparin may be needed as its site of action, antithrombin III, can be greatly reduced in NS. There are no reliable indicators of the risk of thromboembolism to guide prophylaxis. General factors need to be addressed such as immobility from severe oedema, treatment of sepsis, and avoidance of haemoconcentration by excessive diuretic use. Because there is no strong evidence base, there are difficulties in deciding to whom to give prophylactic anticoagulation, and for how long. The factors above (immobility, oedema and haemoconcentration) need to be taken into account, as should the presence of any other pro-coagulant state, but there is no definite 'threshold' of proteinuria or hypoalbuminaemia to signify risk of complications. It is common practice to anticoagulate with heparin and warfarin for as long as the serum albumin is less than 20 g/L with nephrotic-range proteinuria. There will be situations, for example pregnancy, where heparin (typically low molecular weight) alone is used.

Use of prophylactic antibiotics

There are conflicting views on the use of antibiotic and vaccine prophylaxis. There are no trials assessing the use of prophylactic antibiotics in adults. A Cochrane review in 2004 could not recommend any interventions for preventing infections in NS (Wu *et al.*, 2004).

Treatment of NS-associated dyslipidaemia

Hyperlipidaemia is a common feature of NS. Numerous abnormalities in lipids occur including increases in hepatic production of apo B-containing lipoproteins, such as very-low-density lipoproteins (VLDL), low-density lipoproteins (LDL) and lipoprotein(a), as well as alterations in high-density lipoprotein (HDL) levels and impaired removal of cholesterol from the periphery.

There is evidence of increased cardiovascular events in nephrotic patients that could be related to the lipid abnormalities (Ordonez *et al.*, 1993), but as yet no prospective trials show treatment improves survival. There is some evidence from meta-analysis and post-hoc analysis that controlling cholesterol levels improves glomerular function and prevents progression of renal disease in chronic kidney disease, especially those with proteinuria (Sandhu *et al.*, 2006). Thus, it is advisable to treat persistent hyperlipidaemia as one would in the general population. Treating the underlying cause of NS and thereby reducing proteinuria will improve or resolve the dyslipidaemia.

Dietary changes used in NS patients

Muscle wasting is a major problem in severe nephrotic syndrome and patients have a greatly increased albumin turnover. The optimal protein intake for such patients is not clear. A low protein diet runs risks of negative nitrogen balance and arguments can be made for normal or high protein diets.

Salt and water retention are the cause of the oedema in NS. For these reasons it is prudent to salt-restrict NS patients to < 100 mmol sodium per day. Careful judgement of diuretic dose, fluid intake and dietary salt restriction is needed.

Management of primary and secondary glomerular diseases causing NS

The primary glomerular diseases which can cause NS have differing significances for the patient with NS; both in terms of treatment strategy and renal prognosis (a detailed discussion is beyond the scope of this chapter; interested readers are directed to the reference texts in the Further resources section below).

Minimal change nephropathy causing NS has been treated with immunosuppressive agents, primarily corticosteroids, since the 1950s. Over the years, many other agents such as cyclophosphamide, mycophenolate, and calcineurin inhibitors (ciclosporin and tacrolimus) have been used to try to improve responses in steroid-insensitive, frequently-relapsing, or poorly-responding cases. More recherché therapies are beyond the scope of this chapter. There is still no consensus on the treatment of the different causes of the nephrotic syndrome or any definitive answers from randomized controlled trials. Awareness of the use of immunosuppressive agents is very important, as many have significant side-effects (Box 4.5).

Minimal change nephropathy has an excellent prognosis with many patients maintaining their renal function in the long term. The majority of patients respond to a course of corticosteroids; many however can relapse and remain steroid-dependent, sometimes requiring additional agents for achievement of remission.

Focal segmental glomerulosclerosis (FSGS) patients always have nephrotic or non-nephrotic proteinuria. Patients with secondary FSGS have a hyperfiltration injury and should be treated with ACE inhibitors or angiotensin II receptor antagonists. Most untreated patients with primary FSGS will develop chronic kidney disease (CKD) stage 5 from 5 to 20 years after presentation with response to therapy remaining the best prognostic indicator of outcome. Patients often need long courses of high-dose prednisolone, and additional agents, to achieve some remission. Patients who do show remission have a better long-term renal outcome than those who do not.

Membranous nephropathy is an immune mediated glomerular disease associated with malignancy in 7–15% patients over 60 years old. It has a variable renal prognosis. Up to 30% patients remit spontaneously whilst 30% progress to CKD stage 5 within 5–15 years. The best treatment strategy remains controversial especially in view of the high spontaneous remission rates. A Cochrane meta-analysis in 2004 concluded that there was no long-term effect of immunosuppressive treatment on patient and/or renal survival (Schieppati *et al.*, 2004). Most nephrologists feel a trial of immunosuppressive therapy is warranted in patients with idiopathic membranous nephropathy who remain nephrotic despite maximal use of ACE inhibitors and ARB, and in those who have deteriorating renal function.

It is not possible to review all of the evidence for intervention in secondary glomerular pathology leading to NS, but it is noteworthy that, for example, successful intervention to resolve amyloid fibril formation (in both immunocyte- and inflammation-associated amyloidosis) can lead to complete resolution of all proteinuria.

Conclusions

NS is a common condition in nephrological practice and can present in diverse ways in different healthcare settings. It has significant complications. Though one can standardize the investigation and the general management, long-term control of NS remains incomplete, as currently we are unable effectively to combat several primary glomerular diseases that can cause NS. Large randomized trials to

Box 4.5 **Major side-effects of commonly used immunosuppressive agents for nephrotic syndrome**

Immunosuppressive agents all increase the susceptibility to and severity of infection.

Corticosteroids (e.g. prednisolone)
- gastro-intestinal effects;
  - gastritis;
  - ulceration;
- proximal myopathy;
- osteoporosis;
- Cushingoid changes;
- hypertension;
- glucose intolerance.

Cyclophosphamide
- bone marrow depression;
- infection;
- alopecia;
- sterility and effects on reproductive function;
- haemorrhagic cystitis;
- bladder carcinoma;
- nausea and vomiting.

Ciclosporin
- renal impairment (long term);
- hepatic dysfunction;
- tremor;
- hyperkalaemia;
- hypertension;
- hyperlipidaemia;
- gingival hypertrophy.

Tacrolimus
- diabetes mellitus;
- hyperkalaemia;
- hypertension;
- gastro-intestinal disturbances;
- hepatic dysfunction;
- renal impairment.

Mycophenolate mofetil
- leucopenia;
- GI disturbance especially diarrhoea and vomiting.

Other agents
Levamisole:
- gastrointestinal effects.

ascertain the best management of the primary glomerular pathologies responsible for much of NS are overdue.

Further reading

Crew RJ, Radhakrishnan J, Appel G. (2004) Complications of the nephrotic syndrome and their treatment. *Clinical Nephrology*; **62**: 245–59.

Deschênes G, Feraille E, Doucet A. (2003) Mechanisms of oedema in nephrotic syndrome: old theories and new ideas. *Nephrology, Dialysis and Transplantation*; **18**: 454–56.

Gaspari F, Perico N, Remuzzi G. (2006) Timed urine collections are not needed to measure urine protein excretion in clinical practice. *American Journal of Kidney Diseases*; **47** (1): 1–7.

Haas M, Meehan SM, Karrison TG, Spargo BH. (1997) Changing etiologies of unexplained adult nephrotic syndrome: a comparison of renal biopsy findings from 1976–1979 and 1995–1997. *American Journal of Kidney Diseases*; **30**: 621–31.

Hamm LL, Batuman V. (2003) Edema in the nephrotic syndrome: new aspects of an old enigma. *Journal of the American Society of Nephrology*; **14**: 3008–16.

Ichikawa, I., Rennke, H.G., Hoyer, J.R., Badr, K.F., Schor, N., Troy, J.L. *et al.* (1983) Role for intrarenal mechanisms in the impaired salt excretion of experimental nephrotic syndrome. *Journal of Clinical Investigation*; **71**: 91–103.

Koomans, HA. (2003) Pathophysiology of oedema in idiopathic nephrotic syndrome. *Nephrology, Dialysis and Transplantation*; **18** (suppl 6): vi30–vi32.

Korbet SM, Genchi RM, Borok RZ, Schwartz MM. (1996) The racial prevalence of glomerular lesions in nephrotic adults. *American Journal of Kidney Diseases*; **27**: 647–51.

Mees, EJD. (1996) Does it make sense to administer albumin to the patient with nephrotic oedema? *Nephrology, Dialysis and Transplantation*; **11**: 1224–6.

Nakao N, Yoshimura A, Morita H *et al.* (2003) Combination treatment of angiotensin-II receptor blocker and angiotensin-converting-enzyme inhibitor in non-diabetic renal disease (COOPERATE): a randomised controlled trial. *Lancet*; **361**: 117–24.

Nolasco F, Cameron JS, Heywood EF *et al.* (1986) Adult-onset minimal change nephrotic syndrome: a long-term follow-up. *Kidney International*; **29**: 1215–23.

Ogi M, Yokoyama H, Tomosugi N *et al.* (1994) Risk factors for infection and immunoglobulin replacement therapy in adult nephrotic syndrome. *American Journal of Kidney Diseases*; **24**: 427–36.

Ordonez JD, Hiatt RA, Killebrew EJ, Fireman BH. (1993) The increased risk of coronary heart disease associated with nephrotic syndrome. *Kidney International*; **44**: 638–42.

Orth SR, Ritz E. (1998) The nephrotic syndrome. *New England Journal of Medicine*; **338**: 1202–11.

Ruggenenti P, Perusa A, Mosconi L, Pisone R, Remuzzi G. (1998) Urinary protein excretion is the best predictor of ERF in non-diabetic chronic nephropathies. *Kidney International*; **53**: 1209–16.

Sandhu S, Wiebe N, Fried LF, Tonelli M. (2006) Statins for improving renal outcomes: a meta-analysis. *Journal of the American Society of Nephrology*; **17** (7): 2006–16.

Schieppati A, Perna A, Zamora J *et al.* (2004) Immunosuppressive treatment for idiopathic membranous nephropathy in adults with nephrotic syndrome. *Cochrane Database of Systematic Reviews*; **18**: CD004293.

Tsouli SG, Liberopoulos EN, Kiortsis DN, Mikhailidis DP, Elisaf MS. (2006) Combined treatment with angiotensin-converting enzyme inhibitors and angiotensin II receptor blockers: a review of the current evidence. *Journal of Cardiovascular Pharmacology and Therapy*; **11**: 1–15.

Wu HM, Tang JL, Sha ZH, Cao L, Li YP. (2004) Interventions for preventing infection in nephrotic syndrome. *Cochrane Database of Systematic Reviews*; **2**: CD003964.

Further resources

For doctors

Burden R, Tomson C. (2005) Identification, management, and referral of adults with chronic kidney disease: concise guidelines. *Clinical Medicine*; **5**: 635–42. Available online at URL http://www.renal.org/eGFR/eguide.html

Davison AM, Cameron JS, Grünfeld J-P et al. (eds) (2005) *Oxford Textbook of Clinical Nephrology*, 3rd edn. Oxford University Press, Oxford.

Orth SR, Ritz E. (1998) The nephrotic syndrome. *New England Journal of Medicine*; **338**: 1202–11.

Steddon SJ, Ashman N, Cunningham J, Chesser A. (eds) (2006) *Oxford Handbook of Nephrology and Hypertension*. Oxford University Press, Oxford.

For patients

The Renal Unit of the Royal Infirmary of Edinburgh, Scotland, UK (http://renux.dmed.ed.ac.uk/edren/index.html) is an excellent source of information about renal disease for patients and non-specialist practitioners.

The National Kidney Federation UK (http://www.kidney.org.uk). The federation of UK kidney patient groups has a collection of disease resources under the 'Medical information' heading.

CHAPTER 5

Renal Artery Stenosis

Philip Kalra, Satish Jayawardene and David Goldsmith

OVERVIEW

- Renal artery stenosis (RAS) may present as drug-resistant hypertension, acute renal failure (especially with ACE-I or ARB use), chronic renal impairment or recurrent flash pulmonary oedema.
- The most common pointers to clinical diagnosis of RAS are the presence of femoral, renal or aortic bruits and the coexistence of severe extra-renal vascular disease.
- RAS should be considered when marked deterioration in renal function (e.g. >20% increase in creatinine) occurs when an ACE-I or ARB is used.
- Atheromatous renovascular disease (ARVD) is the cause of 90% of cases of RAS, and it can be unilateral or bilateral.
- Postmortem studies indicate the presence of ARVD in over 40% of elderly patients. AVRD does not cause significant hypertension or CKD in the majority of patients.
- Approximately 10% of RAS cases are due to fibromuscular dysplasia (FMD), typically found in hypertensive young women. Angioplasty can cure hypertension in about a third of this group of patients.
- There are several screening methods for RAS.
- Both renal arteriography and angioplasty have significant risks to the patient, which should be considered.
- Renal artery angioplasty and stenting are effective at improving renal artery stenoses for both AVRD and FMD. However, only in FMD can one expect a significant improvement in BP control in the majority of patients.
- AVRD should be considered as part of a diffuse vascular disease process, and management should involve control of hypertension and hyperlipidaemia, use of antiplatelet agents and cessation of smoking.
- Ironically, ACE-I and ARBs are the optimal anti-hypertensive choices for patients with ARVD although care and specialist advice may be necessary if marked renal deterioration is found following the administration of such medication.

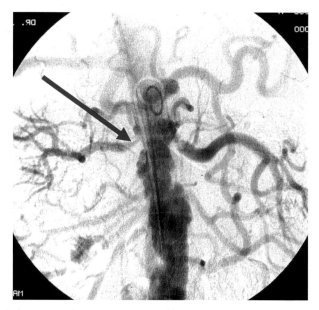

Figure 5.1 Renal arteriogram showing atheromatous renal artery stenosis (RAS). A flush aortogram: note the irregular shape of the aorta due to atheroma. The red arrow points to marked reduction in the arterial lumen of the renal artery. Atheromatous RAS typically involves the ostia of the renal arteries, as these are involved with aortic atherosclerotic lesions.

Definition and background

Renal artery stenosis (RAS) is a reduction in the lumen of one or both renal arteries, and can be an important cause of renal failure and secondary hypertension. In >90% of cases the condition is due to atheroma of the renal arteries (atheromatous renovascular disease, ARVD; Fig. 5.1), and this is a disease of ageing. Patients usually have evidence of atheroma in other important vascular beds, such as coronary artery disease (CAD), cerebrovascular and peripheral vascular disease (PVD), and the RAS involves the renal ostia (renal arterial origins) in 90% of cases. ARVD can be unilateral or bilateral and up to 50% of patients have renal artery occlusion (RAO) at diagnosis. It is very common, postmortem studies indicating its presence in over 40% of elderly patients.

Approximately 5% of RAS cases are due to fibromuscular dysplasia (FMD; Fig. 5.2), which, when it is discovered, is typically seen in hypertensive young women, most of whom have well-preserved renal function. In contrast to ARVD, angioplasty of FMD RAS lesions is usually associated with clinical improvement, such as cure of hypertension in a third of patients.

Although many patients with ARVD will have hypertension and/or chronic kidney disease (CKD), in the vast majority of patients it is likely to be incidental and pathophysiologically insignificant to these latter conditions. This explains the inconsistent results following renal artery intervention in ARVD, which has led to uncertainty

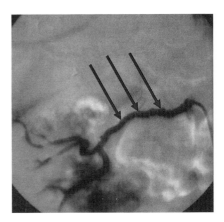

Figure 5.2 Renal arteriogram showing fibromuscular renal artery stenosis (RAS). A selective right renal artery angiogram in fibromuscular RAS (FMD). The aorta is not affected by atheroma. The red arrows point to multiple bead-like irregularities in the lumen of the renal artery well away from the ostium. A nephrogram can be seen, and there is contrast in the renal collecting system and ureter.

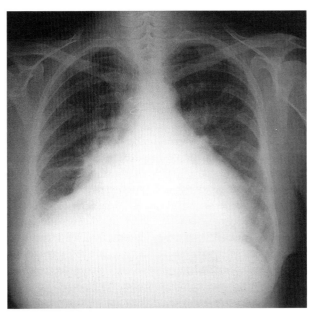

Figure 5.3 'Flash' pulmonary oedema. A chest X-ray which shows florid bilateral pulmonary oedema, which was the presentation of severe RAS in this patient.

in guidelines for its management. Assessing the severity of a stenosis, and a careful understanding of the clinical context, are essential to planning management. Most RAS will be suspected, diagnosed and treated in a hospital setting. One important exception is a change in renal function with the introduction of angiotensin converting enzyme inhibitors (ACE-I) or angiotensin receptor blockers (ARB), as numerically the majority of scripts for hypertension and heart failure are community-based.

Clinical features

Although the majority of ARVD cases are asymptomatic, the condition should be suspected in patients presenting with renal dysfunction and hypertension who have evidence of atheromatous disease in other vascular beds. Particular clinical features include significant deterioration of renal function (e.g. > 20% increase in serum creatinine or fall in eGFR) accompanying use of ACE-I or ARBs, or unexplained 'flash' (sudden onset) pulmonary oedema (Fig. 5.3), but the presence of femoral, renal or aortic bruits and the co-existence of severe extra-renal vascular disease are the commonest clinical pointers to diagnosis. Hypertension may be absent, particularly in patients with chronic cardiac dysfunction, but a high index of suspicion for RAS diagnosis is advised in cases with severe (often systolic) hypertension, especially when unresponsive to three or more anti-hypertensive agents and with evidence of widespread vascular disease. Box 5.1 lists some of the important clinical clues to the presence of RAS.

Pathogenesis of renal dysfunction in patients with RAS

Most interventional treatments for RAS are undertaken with the aim of controlling severe hypertension or reversing, or at least stabilizing, renal dysfunction. In the case of FMD, such treatment is usually justified: here, the hypertension and renal impairment are often

> **Box 5.1 Clinical clues to the presence of RAS**
>
> - Onset of hypertension < 40 years of age.
> - Drug-resistant hypertension.
> - Chronic renal impairment in an atherosclerotic patient.
> - Recurrent flash pulmonary oedema.
> - Widespread arterial disease.
> - Vascular bruits (particularly epigastric and/or renal).
> - Asymmetrical renal size (> 10% difference) on renal ultrasound.
> - Development of significant renal impairment with the introduction of an ACE-I/ARB (20% or more increased creatinine or decreased eGFR).

consequent upon renal ischaemia due to 'hydraulic' effects of the renal arterial narrowing. As the patient is typically young and the kidney beyond the RAS has not been subjected to years of hypertensive and atherosclerotic injury, revascularization can be expected to improve these clinical abnormalities.

However, this is not generally the case with ARVD. There is now compelling evidence that intra-renal injury, probably most often due to long-standing hypertension, dyslipidaemia and inflammation (all of which pre-date RAS development), is the major factor responsible for renal dysfunction in the majority of patients who have CKD with ARVD. Hence, there is often little correlation between severity of RAS and the extent of renal dysfunction in ARVD, and patients with unilateral RAS can develop renal failure even though the contralateral renal artery remains patent. Proteinuria appears to be a key marker of this intra-renal injury and it is strongly linked to baseline renal function as well as long-term outcome. The histological changes of 'ischaemic nephropathy' include a constellation of hypertensive damage, cholesterol athero-embolism, intra-renal vascular disease and sclerosing glomerular lesions. These associations help explain the variable outcomes that occur following renal revascularization procedures, which are discussed later.

Investigations

Screening and diagnostic investigations generally assess relative renal size and renal arterial anatomy, but additional tests (e.g. isotope GFR, which can be used to measure function of individual kidneys) are needed to correlate function with these morphologic parameters. Captopril renography is now rarely used, except perhaps in patients with both severe hypertension and preserved renal function.

Asymmetric renal size (> 1.5 cm difference in bipolar length) at ultrasound is suggestive, but there are many other explanations for such inequality and ARVD is often bilateral. Doppler ultrasonography can be a sensitive screening test but it is time-consuming, highly operator-dependent (and hence not a cost-effective screening tool), and thus only few centres presently offer this facility. Contrast-enhanced CT angiography has an excellent detection rate, but as with conventional intra-arterial angiography (which used to be termed the 'gold standard' investigation for RAS), there is a risk of contrast nephrotoxicity in higher risk patients (e.g. those with GFR < 30 mL/min, diabetics). In high-risk patients radiocontrast procedures should be limited where possible and alternative imaging considered. Intravascular volume depletion is a key risk factor, which can be corrected by appropriate volume expansion with intravenous saline. Oral use of the antioxidant *N*-acetylcysteine has been widely assessed with conflicting results and its role remains uncertain. However, it is an inexpensive agent without significant side-effects and its use in clinical practice may not therefore be inappropriate.

Contrast-enhanced MR angiography (MRA) is becoming the favoured imaging method for the proximal renal vasculature (Fig. 5.4). It is sensitive and gadolinium is non-nephrotoxic at low doses; patient suitability is limited by claustrophobia or by the presence of metallic objects (e.g. aneurysm clips). Recent concerns about fibrosing skin problems seen in patients with advanced CKD and exposure to gadolinium – nephrogenic systemic fibrosis or nephrogenic fibrosing dermopathy (NSF/NFD) – need fuller evaluation. Noteworthy advances in MR techniques include the possibility of measuring

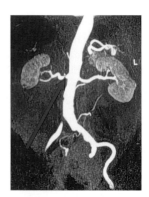

Figure 5.4 Magnetic resonance angiogram showing renal artery stenosis. A magnetic resonance angiogram with intravenous gadolinium contrast enhancement showing aortic irregularity and a tight right renal artery stenosis indicated by the arrow – distally, a smaller kidney compared to the other side.

> **Box 5.2 The management of renal artery stenosis**
>
> - Maximal blood pressure control (may require more than six different anti-hypertensive drugs).
> - Renal artery angioplasty plus stenting for flash pulmonary oedema, severe drug-resistant hypertension, and for preservation of renal function.
> - Statin to reduce hypercholesterolaemia, especially in atherosclerotic RAS.
> - Low-dose aspirin therapy.

individual renal function, with the potential of providing a comprehensive functional and anatomical scan in a single visit.

Management of RAS

In those patients where RAS is an incidental finding with little or no hypertension, no invasive intervention is generally required. As stated previously, renal revascularization, usually with angioplasty alone, is likely to be successful in controlling or even curing hypertension, and in reversing renal dysfunction (when it occurs) in FMD (Box 5.2).

Medical treatment

ARVD should be considered as part of a diffuse vascular disease process rather than as a solitary disease affecting the renal circulation. Extra-renal vascular co-morbidities should not be overlooked, as they may be the major contributor to the poor outcome of ARVD patients. An evidence base to guide best medical 'vascular protective' management is lacking, but attention to limiting the progression of atheromatous disease by control of hypertension and hyperlipidaemia, use of antiplatelet agents and cessation of smoking seem non-controversial approaches. Although it may appear counter-intuitive, both ACE-I and ARBs would be optimal anti-hypertensive choices for patients with ARVD, especially for those with proteinuric chronic parenchymal disease, and those with co-existing CAD and cardiac dysfunction. However, this could only be responsibly undertaken with very careful supervision. In these situations there needs to be a balance between, for example, renal risk and benefit, versus cardiac and cerebral protection. Needless to say, to date no randomized controlled trial has addressed this difficult question.

Renal revascularization

Revascularization procedures have been utilized for the treatment of RAS for over three decades, but percutaneous interventional techniques – angioplasty with/without stent placement (Figs 5.5 and 5.6) – has now largely replaced surgical revascularization, accounting for 95% of all procedures in ARVD. Nevertheless, these procedures should only be performed after careful patient evaluation as complications can occur. Some degree of contrast nephropathy and cholesterol embolization occurs in a large proportion of patients, but they are clinically significant in only a minority; renal arterial rupture or thrombosis are fortunately uncommon. Until now, only four randomized clinical trials have investigated the outcome after

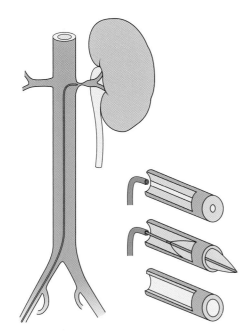

Figure 5.5 Cartoon of renal artery angioplasty.

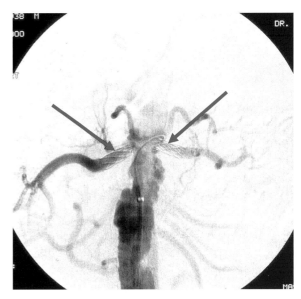

Figure 5.6 Bilateral renal artery stents. A flush aortogram shows the presence of bilateral proximal renal artery stents (the red arrows point to these at the ostia of the renal arteries, just protruding into the aortic lumen).

revascularization in ARVD – none showed any benefit to renal function (but the trials were small and were not adequately powered to do so), but most showed a modest improvement in hypertension control after angioplasty. There are countless retrospective reports from individual centres and in most, irrespective of the revascularization technique, although an improvement in renal function is observed in a minority (< 25%) of patients, the overall effect upon renal functional outcome in the whole ARVD group is generally minimal. Large-scale RCTs are essential to determine the overall effects of intervention, and to help identify which sub-groups of patients will benefit from revascularization. A UK-led international trial, ASTRAL, that will recruit up to 750 patients with ARVD, will be complete in 2007 and will report in 2008.

Despite the uncertainty of the place of renal revascularization in the majority of patients with ARVD, few would dispute its necessity in patients presenting with recurrent 'flash' pulmonary oedema in association with a high grade RAS lesion, as the procedure can be life-saving. There is also reasonable consensus that revascularization should be considered in patients with high-grade RAS and the following clinical scenarios:

- severe hypertension resistant to all medical therapy;
- when a patient who requires ACE-I or ARB therapy (e.g. for cardiac failure) presents with significant ACE-I-related renal dysfunction;
- when there is evidence of recent-onset RAO in a reasonably sized kidney. Such patients present with anuria (if the RAO affects some-

one with a solitary kidney) and rapidly deteriorating renal function. Angioplasty (possibly with prior thrombolytic therapy) can dramatically rescue the functioning renal mass in this situation.

Prognosis of patients with ARVD

Only a minority of patients with CKD and ARVD progress through to need dialysis, the remainder usually dying from cardiovascular complications; a recent US epidemiological study showed that the risk of death of ARVD patients during follow-up was almost six times that of developing ERF. The poor survival relates to patient age but is largely due to the effects of co-morbid cardiovascular disease. In studies from Hope Hospital, ARVD patients have been shown to have a 5-year survival of 52%, but those presenting with ERF had a 30-fold relative risk of mortality compared with patients with well-preserved function; patients with CAD had significantly higher mortality than patients with isolated ARVD.

Further reading

Hegarty J, Wright JR, Kalra PR, Kalra PA. (2006) The heart in renovascular disease – an association demanding further investigation. *Int J Cardiol*; **111**(3): 339–42.

Krumme B, Donauer J. (2006) Atherosclerotic renal artery stenosis and reconstruction. *Kidney Int*; **70**(9):1543–7.

Textor SC. (2006) Renovascular hypertension update. *Curr Hypertens Rep*; **8**(6):521–7.

CHAPTER 6

Urinary Tract Infections, Renal Stones, Renal Cysts and Tumours and Pregnancy in Chronic Kidney Disease

David Goldsmith

OVERVIEW

- Dysuria is usually urinary tract infection-related, but it can be due to urethritis (e.g. chlamydia, herpes) or vaginitis (e.g. *Trichomonas* spp).

- Asymptomatic bacteriuria does not generally need treatment except in pregnancy.

- Pyelonephritis and renal abscesses are potentially life threatening.

- Acute pyelonephritis is suggested by fever, chills, flank pain, fever, raised CRP and white cell count.

- Kidney stones may vary from being asymptomatic, if tiny, to causing colicky loin (often radiating to groin) pain with visible haematuria. The pain may be so severe as to cause vomiting. The risk of infection and obstruction with such cases warrants urgent investigation.

- Kidney stones form in urine that is supersaturated with the chemical constituents. The main types are calcium oxalate, calcium phosphate struvite, urate and cystine.

- Calcium stones are exacerbated by loop diuretics, vitamin D, antacids and steroids, while uric acid stones can be exacerbated by salicylates and are more common in people of Middle Eastern and Mediterranean origin.

- With increased access to renal/abdominal ultrasound and CT scanning, more renal cysts and masses are being discovered incidentally. Any solid renal mass > 3 cm should be regarded as potentially malignant and considered for removal.

- Fertility declines with advancing CKD, pregnancy being very unusual while on dialysis. Successful renal transplantation has a good chance of restoring fertility.

Urinary tract infections in adults

Acute uncomplicated urinary tract infections (UTIs) are one of the most common medical conditions. Their incidence depends on gender, age, sexual activity, and predisposing factors (e.g. urological, anatomical or functional abnormalities, pregnancy, foreign bodies, immunosuppression, host/mucosal immune defences). In sexually active younger women the incidence of cystitis is 0.5 per person-year whereas in adult men aged less than 50 years it is 5–8 episodes per 10 000 men annually. Infections occur when uropathogens (e.g. *Escherichia coli*) present in rectal flora enter the urinary tract via the urethra. More rarely, UTIs occur by haematogenous spread.

Women with uncomplicated UTIs generally present with dysuria, frequency, urgency and suprapubic pain. Dysuria itself of course can

be UTI-related, but can be due to urethritis (e.g. chlamydia, herpes) or vaginitis (*Trichomonas* spp).

In this setting *E. coli* is typically resistant to amoxicillin, and increasing resistance is now being seen to trimethoprim and cotrimoxazole. Trimethoprim is the best first-line option, but it is imperative to be aware of local communities' antibiotic resistance patterns and local hospital/community guidelines. Three-day oral antibiotic courses are preferred (single dose strategies are less effective, but have fewer side-effects). Recurrent episodes are usually due to incomplete eradication rather than re-infection. Women with recurrent cystitis can opt to try altering certain behavioural risk factors (e.g. voiding post-coitus, increasing fluid intake). Cranberry/lingonberry juice (> 200mL/day) can help prevent some UTIs. Antibiotic prophylaxis (e.g. trimethoprim, 200 mg, or cefalexin, 250 mg) can be a highly effective intervention (e.g. regular or post coital) .

Complicated UTIs (e.g. hospital or institution acquired) can be as common as in 5% of hospital admissions (nearly all of these episodes coming from indwelling urinary catheters). Such UTIs are the commonest cause of gram-negative bacteraemias.

Asymptomatic bacteriuria is defined as the presence of two separate clean-voided urine specimens with > 10^5 bacteria/mL of voided urine without symptoms. Five per cent of premenopausal women, and far fewer men, have this. Over the age of 65, around 10% of men and 20% of women have asymptomatic bacteriuria. In pregnancy, treat asymptomatic bacteriuria with amoxicillin, 250–500 mg, thrice-daily for 10 days (or nitrofurantoin if penicillin-allergic).

Aetiologic agents are typically *E. coli* (75–90%) and *S. saprophyticus* (coagulase-negative staphylococcus; 10–20%). *Proteus* spp, *Klebsiella* spp and *Enterobacter* spp are also important, though much more rare.

Acute pyelonephritis is suggested by fever, chills, flank pain, fever, raised CRP and white cell count. Cystitis symptoms are present too. White cells in the urine are ubiquitous unless the infected kidney is also obstructed (e.g. ureteric stone). The kidney is inflamed and oedematous. Parenteral or oral therapy can be chosen, depending on the severity of the infection and other patient-related factors; most cases are dealt with by hospital admission. Fourteen-day courses of potent antibiotics are indicated (e.g. cefuroxime, ciprofloxacin).

Infections that have been caused by the presence of a foreign body, e.g. a urinary catheter, or a ureteric stent, may not improve, or may relapse very early, unless that foreign body is removed, or changed.

Renal abscess is a rare event, e.g. 1–10 per 10 000 hospital admissions. The clinical presentation can be fulminant or indolent. Abscesses can be corticomedullary, peri-renal or cortical (e.g. renal carbuncle in the renal cortex due to *S. aureus*). *Papillary necrosis* is also a rare event, caused by hypoxia in the renal medulla, whose risk factors include age, sickle cell disease or trait (and other haemoglobinopathies), diabetes, analgesic abuse and dehydration. *Papillary necrosis* can cause renal obstruction if the sloughed papillary nubbin lodges in the ureter. *Emphysematous pyelonephritis* is a rare, fulminant necrotizing variant of acute pyelonephritis, often in diabetic patients, and with gas-forming *E. coli, K. pneumoniae, P. mirabilis*; septic peri-nephric haematomata are a complication. *Xanthogranulomatous pyelonephritis* is an even rarer but severe chronic renal infection associated with urinary obstruction. A portion of renal parenchyma is replaced by a dense cellular infiltrate of lipid-laden macrophages; this process can extend outside the kidney. The offending organisms are usually *E. coli* or *S. aureus*.

Kidney stones (nephrolithiasis)

Here, we will discuss only kidney stones (as opposed to stones that form in the bladder or ureter). The main types of renal stone are calcium oxalate, calcium phosphate struvite, urate and cystine. Figures 6.1 and 6.2 shows some renal stones.

Kidney stones can vary from tiny, microscopic deposits with no symptoms to large staghorn calculi filling up the renal pelvis and

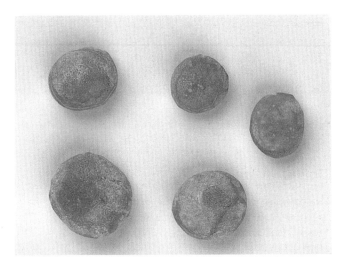

Figure 6.1 Renal stones.

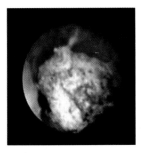

Figure 6.2 Stone obstruction of a ureter (seen at ureterscopy). (Reproduced from *ABC of Urology*, with permission from Blackwell Publishing Ltd.)

Box 6.1 Clinical presentation of kidney stone disease

- Pain (loin to groin, waves, severe)
- Visible haematuria
- Microscopic haematuria
- Infection
- Obstruction

---

causing pain, infection and obstruction. Box 6.1 lists the clinical presentation of kidney stone disease; its severity depends on the stone type, rate of formation, size and location.

Kidney stones are common in industrialized countries, with a peak age of onset in the third decade, and an annual incidence of about 1 in 1000 people. Factors that determine prevalence include age, race, geography, and gender. In the Middle East and Mediterranean countries, uric acid stones can be > 50% of all stones, whereas in the UK they are < 5%. Stone formation can be associated with many different medications – calcium stones with loop diuretics, vitamin D, antacids and steroids; uric acid stones with salicylate and probenecid, and crystalline stones from triamterene, indinivir and aciclovir.

Stones can only form in urine that is supersaturated with the chemical constituents of that stone. Urinary inhibitors of calcification and stone formation (e.g. increased urinary citrate, or a more alkaline urine pH) are also important. Clinical manifestations are typically loin (often radiating to groin) pain (ureteric colic) and visible haematuria. The pain comes in waves and can be excruciatingly severe, causing vomiting.

The basic evaluation of a patient with a renal stone is shown in Box 6.2.

General treatment of renal stones involves relief of pain (preferably using parenteral NSAID or opiates), any urinary obstruction, and infection. Acute surgical intervention may be needed. Prevention of future stone formation or symptomatic episodes is important and is summarized in Box 6.3.

Box 6.2 Basic evaluation of renal stone formers

- Stone history – how many stones, age at first onset, one or both kidneys, need for intervention
- Medical history
- Medications
- Family history
- Physical examination
- Laboratory tests
  - urine – microscopy and culture;
  - pH;
  - stone chemical analysis;
  - urea and electrolytes, chloride, bicarbonate, uric acid, calcium, phosphate;
  - PTH, if calcium elevated.
- Radiological investigations
  - KUB;
  - CT IVU;
  - ultrasound.

Box 6.3 **Prevention of future/recurrent stone formation**

- Increase in fluid intake (to > 2 L/day)
- Limit salt intake (which decreases urinary calcium excretion)
- Increase oral calcium intake (binding dietary oxalate)
- Decrease urinary calcium excretion (thiazide diuretic)
- Reduce dietary oxalate (for oxalate stone formers)

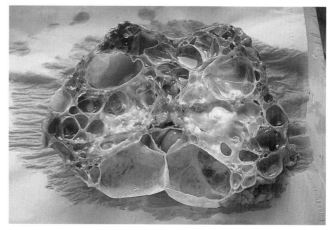

(a)

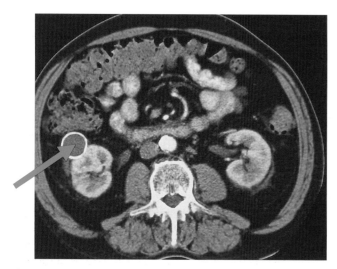

Figure 6.3 Single large calcified renal cyst.

Renal cysts and tumours

In modern hospitals and institutions there is much more ready access to, and use of, renal/abdominal ultrasound and CT scanning. As a result, there are more renal cysts and masses incidentally discovered than before (Fig. 6.3). The key question is the assessment of the risk of malignancy. Ultrasound imaging is only 80% sensitive at detecting renal parenchymal lesions; CT and MRI scanning are much more sensitive techniques. Figure 6.4 shows polycystic kidney disease.

Any solid mass with a diameter > 3 cm should be regarded as potentially malignant and be removed, unless circumstances prevent this. Proximity of a solid renal mass to the renal vein may well determine tumour behaviour as much as the mass's absolute diameter. Mixed solid–cystic lesions present significant difficulties. Causes of renal cystic disease are given in Box 6.4.

Autosomal dominant polycystic kidney disease (ADPKD)

ADPKD, an important cause of hypertension and renal failure in adults, may rarely present in infancy and childhood:

- antenatal ultrasound: discrete cysts in fetal kidneys (although in some people the cysts do not appear until their teens);
- macroscopic haematuria;
- hypertension, renal failure;
- incidental finding of renal cysts during abdominal ultrasound.

ADPKD has no gender or race preference. There may not be a known family history of this condition, and, occasionally, the af-

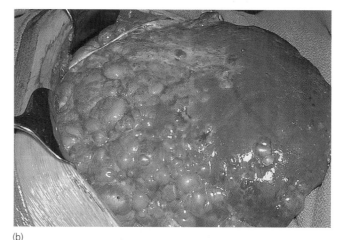

(b)

Figure 6.4 Polycystic kidney disease: (a) kidney and (b) cysts in liver.

Box 6.4 **Renal cystic diseases**

Non-genetic
- simple cysts (increasingly common in those aged > 50 years);
- medullary sponge kidney;
- medullary cystic disease;
- acquired multi-cystic disease (in advanced CKD).

Genetic
- autosomal dominant polycystic disease (mostly adults);
- Von Hippel Lindau disease;
- tubero-sclerosis;
- autosomal recessive polycystic disease (mostly children);
- nephronophthisis;
- multicystic/dysplastic syndromes.

fected parent is only diagnosed by ultrasound performed after the condition is detected in their child. See also Fig. 6.4b (cysts are seen in the liver in 50% of patients).

ADPKD can cause cysts in the liver and problems in other organs, such as the heart and blood vessels in the brain. In the United States, about 500 000 people have ADPKD, and it is the fourth leading cause of kidney failure.

ADPKD is one of the most common inherited disorders. The phrase 'autosomal dominant' means that if one parent has the disease, there is a 50% chance that the disease will pass to a child. Either the mother or father can pass it on, but new mutations may account for a quarter of new cases.

Many people with ADPKD live for decades without developing symptoms. For this reason, ADPKD is often called 'adult polycystic kidney disease'.

Symptoms of ADPKD

The most common symptoms are pain in the back and the sides (between the ribs and hips), and headaches. The dull pain can be temporary or persistent, mild or severe.

People with ADPKD can also experience the following:
- urinary tract infections;
- haematuria;
- liver and pancreatic cysts;
- abnormal heart valves;
- high blood pressure;
- kidney stones;
- cerebral and other aneurysms;
- diverticulosis.

Diagnosis of ADPKD

To diagnose ADPKD, the ultrasound should show three or more kidney cysts. Typically there are many more than this, in enlarged kidneys, and the cysts often distort the shape of the kidney as well as cause it to enlarge. The diagnosis is strengthened by a family history of ADPKD, and the presence of cysts in other organs.

Once the condition is established in one family member, it is good practice to offer to screen other family members too. In the case of children (< 15 years old), a normal ultrasound scan cannot guarantee that there is no ADPKD and so it is not recommended to screen children until they have reached early adulthood – the cysts can develop and become manifest only in adult life. It is very unusual however for a normal screening ultrasound to be falsely negative (or normal) with a subject aged > 20 years.

A genetic test can detect mutations in the PKD1 and PKD2 genes. Although this test can detect the presence of the ADPKD mutations before cysts develop, its usefulness is limited by two factors: it cannot predict the onset or ultimate severity of the disease, and no absolute cure is available to prevent the onset of the disease. On the other hand, a young person who knows of an ADPKD gene mutation may be able to forestall the disease through diet and blood pressure control. The test may also be used to determine whether a young member of an ADPKD family can safely donate a kidney to a parent. Anyone considering genetic testing should receive counselling to understand all the implications of the test.

Treatment of ADPKD

Although a cure for ADPKD is not yet available, treatment can ease the symptoms and prolong life. Novel therapies are also soon to be clinically available.

Renal, back and cyst pain

These can be caused by kidney stones, urinary tract infections, cyst infection or cyst haemorrhage. Therapies include bed rest and antibiotics, and much more rarely, cyst aspiration under ultrasound or CT guidance. High blood pressure is very common indeed in ADPKD, though keeping BP under control unfortunately has little effect on the progression of ADPKD.

Pregnancy in CKD

Pregnancy may be the first time that young women have their BP checked, or urine tests performed, so a small number of pregnant women are discovered to have haematuria, proteinuria, pyuria, raised BP or renal impairment.

Microscopic haematuria can be detected in up to 25% of normal pregnancies at some stage. This disappears in the majority after delivery. Causes include glomerular disease, pre-eclampsia, and urinary tract infection. Macroscopic haematuria is rare, and most often due to urine infection.

The development of significant proteinuria during pregnancy always requires evaluation and investigation. Up to 95% of pregnant women excrete less than 200 mg protein/24 h. A protein:creatinine ratio > 30 mg protein/mmol creatinine is abnormal (i.e. the upper limit of normal for PCR is 30 in pregnancy compared to 15 in the non-pregnant state). Persistent *de novo* proteinuria in pregnancy is most often due to pre-eclampsia, when raised BP is typically seen in the second half of pregnancy. Significant proteinuria in pre-eclampsia confers a higher risk of adverse maternal and foetal outcome. Proteinuria due to pre-eclampsia should resolve within a few months of delivery, so persistent proteinuria suggests that pregnancy has unmasked prior renal disease.

There is no specific treatment for proteinuria in pregnancy; ACEI and ARB are contra-indicated because of unwanted fetal side-effects. If the pregnant woman becomes nephrotic there is a direct relationship between maternal plasma albumin and birth weight. Renal biopsy can safely be performed in pregnancy, and depending on the result, specific treatment, including immunosuppression, can be considered.

Asymptomatic bacteriuria affects 2–10% of all women and can lead to serious complications in pregnancy (acute pyelonephritis, and sometimes premature delivery), so is worth screening for (urine dipstick/nitrites, then culture if positive) and treating (amoxicillin/clavulinic acid, nitrofurantoin or second generation cephalosporin). It is more common in women with urological anatomical or functional abnormalities, diabetic women, and older multiparous women. The overall incidence of pyelonephritis in pregnancy is approximately 1% (usually second trimester), but amongst women with asymptomatic bacteriuria can be as high as 25%.

Acute renal failure in pregnancy was a feature of around 1 in 2000 pregnancies in the 1960s; the commonest reasons being septic abortion, or in the third trimester obstetric haemorrhage or eclampsia. ARF requiring dialysis in the modern era is much rarer; causes include antepartum haemorrhage, pre-eclampsia, urinary obstruction, sepsis and haemolytic-uraemic syndrome. Rapid restoration of circulating volume (if depleted) is vital for maternal and fetal outcome.

Fertility rapidly declines with advancing CKD, so few women with significant reduction of renal function become pregnant; there is an increased rate of fetal loss, and early delivery is more common in established CKD. Renal function can worsen irreversibly with pregnancy. Pregnancy while on dialysis is very unusual indeed, and delivery of a live infant is truly exceptional. Significant proteinuria, and starting pregnancy with abnormal renal function, are bad prognostic (foetal and maternal renal function) features. Renal transplantation, if successful, can restore fertility and the chance of successful delivery; prednisolone azathioprine, mycophenolate, ciclosporin and tacrolimus are safe drugs to take in pregnancy (though breast feeding is often not recommended because of entry of these drugs into breast milk). Other newer immunosuppressants require more extensive research before we can be certain of their safety profiles.

Further reading

Bisceglia M, Galliani CA, Senger C, Stallone C, Sessa A. (2006) Renal cystic diseases: a review. *Adv Anat Pathol*; **13**(1):26–56.

Stratta P, Canavese C, Quaglia M. (2006) Pregnancy in patients with kidney disease. *J Nephrol*; **19**(2):135–43.

Sutters M. (2006) The pathogenesis of autosomal dominant polycystic kidney disease. *Nephron Exp Nephrol*; **103**(4):e149–55.

Taylor EN, Curhan GC. (2006) Diet and fluid prescription in stone disease. *Kidney Int*; **70**(5):835–9.

CHAPTER 7

Acute Kidney Injury

Rachel Hilton

OVERVIEW

- The term acute kidney injury (AKI) is now preferred in kidney circles to the older term acute renal failure (ARF), but we retain the use of ARF in this chapter for ease of recognition by non-nephrological readers

- The life-threatening consequences of ARF are volume overload, hyperkalaemia and metabolic acidosis.

- ARF is more common in the elderly and those with underlying chronic kidney disease.

- Precipitating factors include: hypovolaemia and hypotension (pre-renal); the use of nephrotoxic drugs and radiographic contrast (intrinsic renal); and obstruction from e.g. stones, malignancy or retroperitoneal fibrosis (post-renal).

- Prevention strategies include maintaining adequate blood pressure, ensuring adequate volume status, and avoiding potentially nephrotoxic drugs.

- ARF is frequently reversible, and rapid recognition and treatment may prevent irreversible nephron loss.

- If past creatinine measurements are not available, useful differentiating features of acute as opposed to chronic renal failure may be the absence of anaemia, hypocalcaemia, hyperphosphataemia and/or reduced renal size and cortical thickness, which often accompany chronic renal failure.

- Acute tubular necrosis is the commonest cause of intrinsic renal disease, and if the precipitating factor has been removed or treated, prognosis is generally good. However, other causes must always be excluded as they have important management implications:
  - rashes, arthralgia or myalgia might suggest an underlying multi-system disease;
  - antibiotics or NSAIDs may cause interstitial nephritis;
  - microscopic haematuria or proteinuria, or dysmorphic red cells or red cell casts, may suggest renal inflammation such as glomerulonephritis or acute interstitial nephritis.

Definition and classification

Acute renal failure (ARF) is characterized by a rapid fall in glomerular filtration rate (GFR), clinically manifest as an abrupt and sustained rise in urea and creatinine. Potentially life-threatening consequences include volume overload, hyperkalaemia and metabolic acidosis. The recently developed RIFLE criteria classify ARF according to degree and outcome (Fig. 7.1).

Epidemiology

ARF is increasingly common: this probably reflects true increased incidence, and also better detection. Recent data suggest an incidence of ARF, defined as serum creatinine above 500 μmol/L, of around 500 per million population (pmp) per year, which is twice the UK prevalence of haemodialysis patients and therefore places high demands upon healthcare resources. ARF is more common with increasing age, the highest incidence being in the 80–89 year age group (950 pmp/year).

ARF complicates at least 5% of hospital admissions, mostly in patients with underlying chronic kidney disease, and is generally multifactorial, chiefly associated with hypovolaemia, hypotension and the use of nephrotoxic drugs or radiographic contrast. When severe enough to require dialysis, in-hospital mortality is around 50%, and may exceed 75% in the context of sepsis or in the critically ill.

Aetiology

The causes of ARF can be grouped into three major categories (Fig. 7.2):

- decreased renal blood flow (pre-renal; 40–80% of cases);
- direct renal parenchymal damage (intrinsic renal; 35–40% of cases);
- obstructed urine flow (post-renal or obstructive; 2–10% of cases).

Pre-renal ARF

Renal blood flow (RBF) and GFR remain roughly constant over a wide range of mean arterial pressures due to changes in afferent (pre-glomerular) and efferent (post-glomerular) arteriolar resistance. Below 70 mmHg, autoregulation is impaired and GFR falls proportionately. Renal autoregulation chiefly depends on a combination of afferent arteriolar vasodilatation mediated by prostaglandins and nitric oxide, and efferent arteriolar vasoconstriction mediated by angiotensin II. Drugs that interfere with these mediators may provoke pre-renal ARF (Table 7.1) in certain settings. With renal artery stenosis or volume depletion, GFR maintenance is particularly angiotensin II-dependent and use of angiotensin converting enzyme (ACE) inhibitors or angiotensin II receptor antagonists can induce

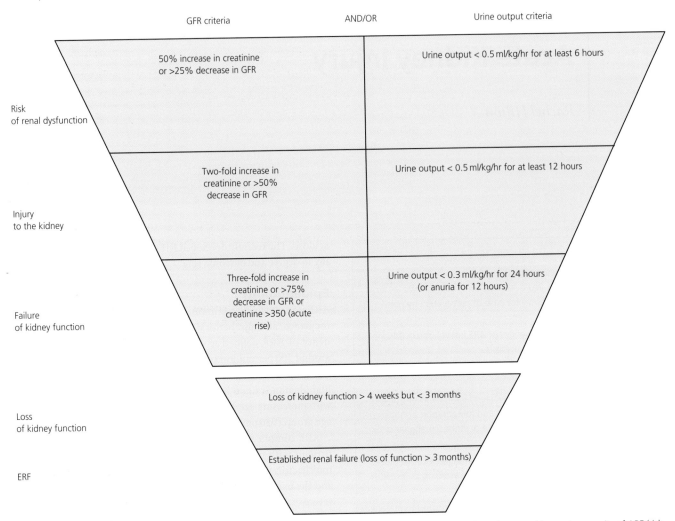

GFR criteria   AND/OR   Urine output criteria

Risk of renal dysfunction — 50% increase in creatinine or >25% decrease in GFR — Urine output < 0.5 ml/kg/hr for at least 6 hours

Injury to the kidney — Two-fold increase in creatinine or >50% decrease in GFR — Urine output < 0.5 ml/kg/hr for at least 12 hours

Failure of kidney function — Three-fold increase in creatinine or >75% decrease in GFR or creatinine >350 (acute rise) — Urine output < 0.3 ml/kg/hr for 24 hours (or anuria for 12 hours)

Loss of kidney function — Loss of kidney function > 4 weeks but < 3 months

ERF — Established renal failure (loss of function > 3 months)

Figure 7.1 Acute renal failure (ARF) classified according to degree and outcome by RIFLE criteria. RIFLE defines three degrees of increasing severity of ARF (risk, injury and failure) and two possible outcomes (loss and ERF).

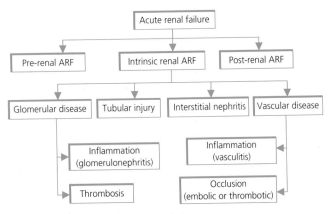

Figure 7.2 Aetiology. ARF: acute renal failure.

ARF. With volume depletion angiotensin II and noradrenaline levels are generally high, and in this setting NSAIDs or cyclooxygenase (COX) inhibitors, which inhibit prostaglandin synthesis, permit unopposed action of local vasoconstrictors on both afferent and efferent arterioles leading to an acute decline in GFR.

Intrinsic renal ARF

Parenchymal causes of ARF may be subdivided into those primarily affecting the glomeruli, the tubules, the intra-renal vasculature, or the renal interstitium. Overall, the commonest cause is acute tubular necrosis (ATN) (Figs 7.3 and 7.4), resulting from continuation of the same pathophysiological processes that lead to pre-renal hypoperfusion. In intensive care the commonest cause is sepsis, frequently accompanied by multi-organ failure. Post-operative ATN accounts for up to 25% of cases of hospital-acquired ARF, mostly due to pre-renal causes. The third commonest cause of hospital-acquired ARF is acute radiocontrast nephropathy. See also Table 7.2.

Post-renal ARF

Obstructive nephropathy presents as ARF relatively infrequently, but rapid diagnosis by ultrasound and prompt intervention to relieve obstruction can result in improvement or even complete recovery of renal function. An important clinical consequence is the substantial diuresis that generally occurs once obstruction is relieved, which

Table 7.1 Principal causes of pre-renal acute renal failure (ARF)

Hypovolaemia	Hypotension	Renal hypoperfusion	Oedema states
Haemorrhage	Cardiogenic shock	Reduced renal perfusion plus impaired autoregulation (e.g. hypovolaemia plus NSAID/COX2 inhibitor or ACE inhibitor/angiotensin II receptor antagonist)	Cardiac failure
GI losses (e.g. vomiting, diarrhoea)	Distributive shock (e.g. sepsis, anaphylaxis)	Abdominal aortic aneurysm	Hepatic cirrhosis
Urinary losses (e.g. glycosuria, post-obstructive diuresis, diuretics)		Renal artery stenosis/occlusion	Nephrotic syndrome (particularly minimal change nephropathy)
Cutaneous losses (e.g. burns)		Hepatorenal syndrome	
Fluid redistribution (e.g. GI obstruction, pancreatitis)			

GI: gastrointestinal; NSAID: nonsteroidal anti-inflammatory drug; COX2: Cyclooxygenase; ACE: angiotension converting enzyme.

Table 7.2 Principal causes of intrinsic renal acute renal failure (ARF)

Glomerular disease	Tubular injury	Interstitial nephritis	Vascular
Inflammatory: e.g. post-infectious glomerulonephritis, cryoglobulinaemia, Henoch–Schönlein purpura, SLE, ANCA-associated glomerulonephritis, anti-GBM disease	Ischaemia: prolonged renal hypoperfusion	Drug-induced: e.g. NSAIDs, antibiotics	Vasculitis (usually ANCA-associated)
Thrombotic: e.g. DIC (Fig. 7.5), thrombotic microangiopathy	Toxins: drugs (e.g. aminoglycosides), radiocontrast, pigments (e.g. myoglobin), heavy metals (e.g. cisplatinum)	Infiltrative: e.g. lymphoma	Cryoglobulinaemia
	Metabolic: hypercalcaemia, immunoglobulin light chains	Granulomatous: sarcoidosis, TB	Polyarteritis nodosa
	Crystals: e.g. urate, oxalate	Infection-related: e.g. post-infective; pyelonephritis	Thrombotic microangiopathy
			Cholesterol emboli
			Renal artery or renal vein thrombosis

SLE; ANCA: antineutrophil cytoplasmic antibody; GBM: glomerular basement membrane; DIC: disseminated intravascular coagulation; NSAID: nonsteroidal anti-inflammatory drugs; TB: tuberculosis.

requires careful monitoring and appropriate fluid replacement to avoid volume depletion. See also Table 7.3.

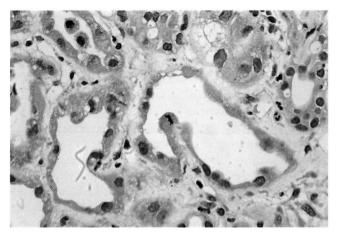

Figure 7.3 A histological view of renal tubular dilatation and loss of renal tubular epithelial cells in acute renal failure ('acute tubular necrosis').

Prevention

The key preventative strategy is to identify patients most at risk, including the elderly, patients with diabetes, hypertension or vascular disease, and those with pre-existing renal impairment. Appropriate preventative measures include maintenance of adequate blood pressure and volume status and avoidance of potentially nephrotoxic agents, particularly NSAIDs, ACE inhibitors or angiotension-II-receptor blockers, as discussed earlier. Among the many causes of ARF, radiocontrast nephropathy is potentially preventable. In high-risk patients, radiocontrast procedures should be limited where possible and alternative imaging considered. Intravascular volume depletion is a key risk factor, which can be corrected by appropriate volume expansion with intravenous saline. Oral use of the antioxidant *N*-acetylcysteine has been widely assessed with conflicting results and its role remains uncertain. However, it is an inexpensive agent without significant side-effects and its use in clinical practice may therefore be appropriate.

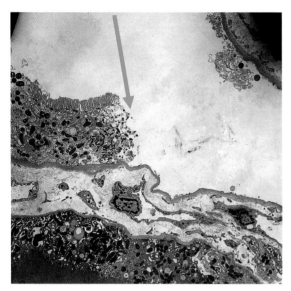

Figure 7.4 Electron micrograph of disrupted renal tubilar epithelium in acute tubular necrosis. The arrow points to the segment where the delicate microvillous tubular epithelial lining is lost

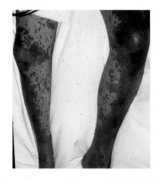

Figure 7.5 Disseminated intravascular coagulation (DIC).

Table 7.3 Principal causes of post-renal acute renal failure (ARF)

Intrinsic	Extrinsic
Intra-luminal: e.g. stone, blood clot, papillary necrosis	Pelvic malignancy
Intra-mural: e.g. urethral stricture, prostatic hypertrophy or malignancy, bladder tumour, radiation fibrosis	Retroperitoneal fibrosis

Differential diagnosis

ARF is frequently reversible and rapid recognition and treatment may prevent irreversible nephron loss. The diagnostic approach to the patient with ARF involves a careful history, including scrutiny of the case notes and drug chart, thorough physical examination and interpretation of appropriate investigations including laboratory tests and imaging (Fig. 7.6).

Is this acute or chronic renal failure?

In this respect, much useful information may be gleaned from the patient notes, from previous biochemistry reports and from GP records, which may save a great deal of unnecessary investigation. Clues from the history and examination include evidence of long-standing diabetes and/or hypertension, though uraemic symptoms in themselves may be modest and/or non-specific. Anaemia, hypocalcaemia and hyperphosphataemia are typical of chronic renal failure but not universal. The most useful clue comes from previous creatinine measurements, if these can be found. Reduced renal size and cortical thickness on ultrasound is a feature of chronic renal failure, although renal size is generally preserved in patients with diabetes.

Has obstruction been excluded?

Careful urological evaluation is mandatory if the cause of ARF is not otherwise apparent, and this includes enquiry about previous stones or symptoms of bladder outflow obstruction and palpation for a palpable bladder. Anuria is an important clue, as this is otherwise unusual in ARF. Renal ultrasound is the method of choice to detect dilatation of the renal pelvis and calyces, although obstruction may be present without dilatation, particularly in cases of malignancy.

Is the patient euvolaemic?

Intravascular volume depletion is indicated by low venous pressure and a postural fall in blood pressure, whereas volume overload manifests as raised venous pressure and pulmonary crepitations. Circumstances leading to pre-renal ARF are almost invariably associated with high levels of plasma antidiuretic hormone, leading to increased tubular reabsorption of both water and urea and a disproportional increase in the plasma urea:creatinine ratio. However, plasma urea may also be raised in the setting of increased catabolism due for example to sepsis or corticosteroid therapy, or protein load due for example to upper GI bleeding. Typically, in pre-renal ARF there is avid retention of sodium and water leading to low urinary sodium concentration. In clinical practice however, the use of diuretics frequently renders urinary indices uninterpretable. If doubt remains, a fluid challenge should be undertaken, but under continuous medical observation (JVP, BP, urine volume) as life-threatening pulmonary oedema may be induced, particularly if the patient is oliguric or anuric (Fig. 7.7).

Is there evidence of renal parenchymal disease (other than ATN)?

Intrinsic renal disease other than ATN is uncommon, but must always be excluded as this has important management implications. The history and examination may suggest an underlying multi-system disease and it is helpful to ask specifically about rashes, arthralgia or myalgia. A careful drug history enquiring specifically about use of antibiotics and NSAIDs (widely available without prescription) is essential, as these commonly used drugs can cause acute interstitial nephritis. Urine dipstick and microscopy are mandatory to avoid missing a renal inflammatory process. Urinary catheterization can cause haematuria, and the concentrated urine seen in ARF can be rich in casts. The presence of significant blood or protein on dipstick (3+/4+), or dysmorphic red cells, red cell casts (suggestive of glomerulonephritis) or eosinophils (suggestive of acute interstitial nephritis) on microscopy – assuming that competent

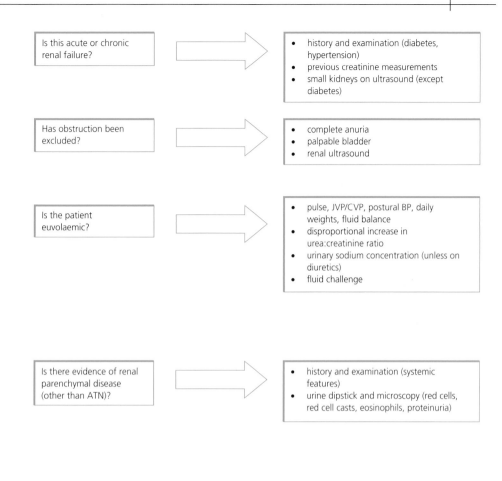

Is this acute or chronic renal failure?

- history and examination (diabetes, hypertension)
- previous creatinine measurements
- small kidneys on ultrasound (except diabetes)

Has obstruction been excluded?

- complete anuria
- palpable bladder
- renal ultrasound

Is the patient euvolaemic?

- pulse, JVP/CVP, postural BP, daily weights, fluid balance
- disproportional increase in urea:creatinine ratio
- urinary sodium concentration (unless on diuretics)
- fluid challenge

Is there evidence of renal parenchymal disease (other than ATN)?

- history and examination (systemic features)
- urine dipstick and microscopy (red cells, red cell casts, eosinophils, proteinuria)

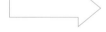

Has a major vascular occlusion occurred?

- atherosclerotic vascular disease
- renal asymmetry
- loin pain
- macroscopic haematuria
- complete anuria

Figure 7.6 Differential diagnosis. JVP: Jugular venous pressure; CVP: central venous pressure ; BP: blood pressure; ATN: acute tubular necrosis.

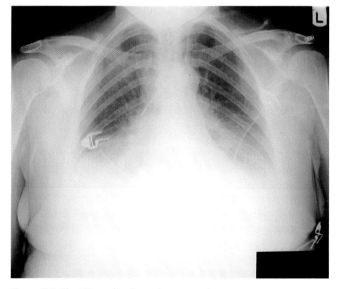

Figure 7.7 Chest X-ray showing pulmonary oedema.

urinary microscopy is available – warrants prompt referral to a nephrologist.

Has a major vascular occlusion occurred?

ARF is common in the elderly, as is co-existent atherosclerotic vascular disease that frequently involves the renal arteries. Whereas occlusion of a normal renal artery results in loin pain and haematuria, occlusion of a previously stenosed renal artery may be clinically silent, leaving the patient dependent upon a single functioning kidney. An important clue is renal asymmetry on imaging, particularly in a patient with vascular disease elsewhere. In this setting, ARF may be precipitated by occlusion (thrombotic or embolic) of the artery supplying the remaining kidney. Risk factors include use of ACE inhibitors and diuretics in the context of renal artery stenosis, hypotension (either drug-induced or due to volume depletion), or instrumentation of the renal artery or aorta. The diagnosis is supported by the presence of complete anuria. Occlusion of a previously normal renal artery is relatively rare, most commonly arising as a consequence of embolization from a central source.

Table 7.4 Scheme of investigation

	Test	Comments
Urinalysis	Dipstick for blood and/or protein	Suggestive of a renal inflammatory process
	Microscopy for cells, casts, crystals	Red cell casts diagnostic in glomerulonephritis
Biochemistry	Serial urea, creatinine, electrolytes Blood gas analysis, serum bicarbonate	Important metabolic consequences of acute renal failure include hyperkalaemia, metabolic acidosis, hypocalcaemia, hyperphosphataemia
	Creatine kinase, myoglobinuria	Markedly elevated creatine kinase and myoglobinuria suggestive of rhabdomyolysis (Fig. 7.8)
	C-reactive protein	Non-specific marker of infection or inflammation
	Serum immunoglobulins, serum protein electrophoresis, Bence Jones proteinuria	Immune paresis, monoclonal band on serum protein electrophoresis and Bence Jones proteinuria suggestive of myeloma
Haematology	Full blood count, blood film	Eosinophilia may be present in acute interstitial nephritis, cholesterol embolization or vasculitis Thrombocytopenia and red cell fragments suggestive of thrombotic microangiopathy
	Coagulation studies	Disseminated intravascular coagulation associated with sepsis
Immunology	Anti-nuclear antibody (ANA) Anti-double-stranded DNA antibodies	ANA positive in systemic lupus erythematosus (SLE) and other autoimmune disorders; anti-dsDNA antibodies more specific for SLE
	Antineutrophil cytoplasmic antibody (ANCA) Antiproteinase 3 (PR3) antibodies Antimyeloperoxidase (MPO) antibodies	Associated with systemic vasculitis c-ANCA and anti-PR3 antibodies associated with Wegener's granulomatosis; p-ANCA and anti-MPO antibodies present in microscopic polyangiitis
	Complement levels	Low in SLE, acute post-infectious glomerulonephritis, essential cryoglobulinaemia
	Antiglomerular basement membrane antibodies	Present in Goodpasture's disease
	Antistreptolysin O and anti-DNAse B titres	Elevated following streptococcal infection
Virology	Hepatitis B and C; HIV	Important implications for infection control within the dialysis area
Radiology	Renal ultrasound	Gives important information about renal size, symmetry, evidence of obstruction

Investigations

A scheme of investigation is shown in Table 7.4, though clearly this should be tailored to individual circumstances. It is unnecessary, for example, to request a full battery of immunological tests in a patient with post-operative ATN or urinary tract obstruction, but this is appropriate if the diagnosis is uncertain or a renal inflammatory condition is suspected (e.g. in the setting of proteinuria and/or haematuria).

Management principles

Management of established ARF encompasses general measures irrespective of cause (Box 7.1) and specific therapies targeted to the particular aetiology, the latter being beyond the scope of this chapter. No pharmacological therapy has been shown to limit the progression of or speed up the recovery from ARF, and indeed some drugs may be harmful (Table 7.5).

Summary

ARF is common and carries a high mortality rate. It is crucial to identify at-risk patients and institute appropriate preventative meas-

ures. Management of ARF includes prevention of life-threatening metabolic consequences, and early referral to a nephrologist where appropriate.

Box 7.1 **Management principles in acute renal failure**

- Identify and correct pre-renal and post-renal factors.
- Optimize cardiac output and renal blood flow.
- Review medication: cease nephrotoxic agents; adjust doses where appropriate; monitor levels where appropriate.
- Accurately monitor fluid intake and output and daily body-weight.
- Identify and treat acute complications (hyperkalaemia, acidosis, hyperphosphataemia, pulmonary oedema).
- Optimize nutritional support: adequate calories but minimize nitrogenous waste production; potassium restriction (Fig. 7.9).
- Identify and aggressively treat infection; minimize indwelling lines; remove bladder catheter if anuric.
- Identify and treat bleeding tendency (Fig. 7.10): prophylaxis with proton pump inhibitor or H_2-antagonist; transfuse if required; avoid aspirin.
- Initiate dialysis before uraemic complications emerge.

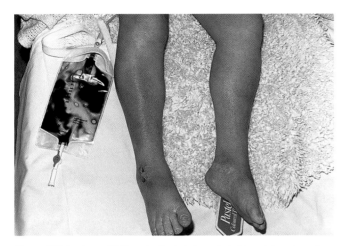

Figure 7.8 Acute renal failure due to rhabdomyolysis (chocolate coloured urine can be seen in the catheter bag).

Table 7.5 Treatment of ARF

Treatment	Evidence of benefit	Comment
Loop diuretics	No difference in renal recovery or mortality compared with placebo	May promote diuresis in oliguric ARF, but may be ototoxic in high doses
Dopamine	No difference in mortality or need for dialysis compared with placebo	Potential adverse effects include tachycardia, extravasation necrosis and peripheral gangrene
Natriuretic peptides	No difference in dialysis-free survival compared with placebo	
Renal replacement therapy	No significant difference in dialysis-dependency or mortality between continuous and intermittent renal replacement therapy	Continuous renal replacement therapy is less likely to provoke haemodynamic instability

Further reading

Allen A. (2002) The aetiology of acute renal failure. In: Glynne P, Allen A, Pusey

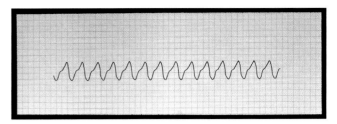

Figure 7.9 An ECG showing sinusoidal waves, in an acute renal failure patient with a plasma potassium of 7.9 mmol/L.

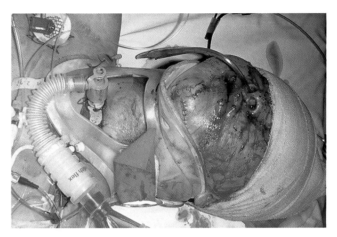

Figure 7.10 A trauma victim: massive exsanguination can lead to acute kidney injury.

CD. (eds) *Acute Renal Failure in Practice*, pp. 39–45. Imperial College Press, London.

Firth JD. (2005) The clinical approach to the patient with acute renal failure. In: Davison AM, Cameron JS, Grunfeld J-P *et al.* (eds) *Oxford Texbook of Clinical Nephrology*, 3rd edn, pp. 1465–1493. Oxford University Press, Oxford.

Kellum, JA. Treating acute renal failure: a guide to the evidence. Available at URL http://www.bmjlearning.com

Lameire N, Van Biesen W, Vanholder R. (2005) Acute renal failure. *Lancet* **365**, 417–430.

CHAPTER 8

Chronic Kidney Disease, Dialysis and Transplantation in Children

Judy Taylor, Christopher Reid

OVERVIEW

Congenital and structural renal disease

- Antenatal ultrasound scanning during pregnancy detects a range of structural renal abnormalities which require assessment and follow up during infancy.
- Urinary tract infection is commoner in infants in children with certain structural abnormalities of the urinary tract.
- Congenital renal dysplasia is the commonest cause of renal failure in childhood.
- Genetically inherited renal diseases are most likely to present in childhood. These include autosomal recessive polycystic kidney disease, Alport's syndrome, and several rare tubular and metabolic disorders.

Childhood nephrotic syndrome

- In nephrotic syndrome, the glomeruli allow small proteins such as albumin to leak out into the urine.
- Childhood nephrotic syndrome commonly occurs between the ages of 1 and 5 years, in boys more often than in girls.
- The majority of children (80–85%) are responsive to steroid treatment, though many of these will have a relapsing course. Other immunosuppressive therapy may be indicated in children who relapse frequently, to minimize the side-effects of steroids.
- Most children 'outgrow' nephrotic syndrome by their late teens without permanent damage to their kidneys, and have an excellent long-term prognosis.
- Renal biopsy is normally reserved for those who do not respond to steroid treatment. In these children, focal segmental glomerulosclerosis is the commonest histological diagnosis with a much poorer prognosis.

Glomerulonephritis

- Glomerulonephritis is an inflammation of the glomeruli and may be temporary and reversible, or it may progress of chronic renal failure. It is usually manifest by raised blood pressure, microscopic haematuria, proteinuria and renal impairment.
- Acute post-streptococcal glomerulonephritis is the commonest cause, with an excellent prognosis for recovery.
- Henoch–Schönlein Purpura is frequently associated with renal involvement, though this is usually clinically mild and self-limiting. A minority may develop severe glomerulonephritis.
- Haemolytic uraemic syndrome is the commonest cause of acute renal failure in childhood. Full recovery is usual when associated with E. coli 0157 enterocolitis and diarrhoea.

Renal replacement therapy

- In infants with renal failure, difficult vascular access and inherent cardiovascular instability means that peritoneal dialysis, as opposed to haemodialysis, is usually the modality of choice.
- Transplantation (usually possible from around 2 years of age) offers the best quality of life even though re-grafting is probably inevitable at some stage.
- Living related donor transplantation is increasingly undertaken in most paediatric centres, and this facilitates pre-emptive transplantation whereby dialysis is avoided.

Introduction

Although many of the principles governing kidney disease management are common to adults and children, the underlying disease spectrum is very different, and children are more than just 'small adults' when it comes to diagnosis and treatment. In this chapter, we will therefore concentrate on conditions which are specific to children or where there are particular issues relating to the diseases in childhood.

Structural abnormalities of the kidneys and urinary tract

These are commonly detected antenatally (Table 8.1), usually at the 20-week anomaly scan, or in early childhood, often with urinary tract infection (UTI). Some simple examples of congenital urogenital abnormalities are shown in Figure 8.1. Some presentations of UTI are shown in Table 8.2.

Renal pelvic dilatation (RPD)

This is the most common finding. A fetal renal pelvis of $>5\,mm$ in the anteroposterior diameter is generally considered abnormal, especially if it progresses on serial scans. A common approach is to start prophylactic trimethoprim at birth and perform ultrasound scans at 1 and 6 weeks after birth. If both are normal, then the infant needs no further investigation and prophylaxis can be stopped;

Table 8.1 Antenatal abnormalities of kidneys and urinary tract

Diagnosis	Features on antenatal scan
Obstruction:	
PUJ	Renal pelvic dilation +/– calyceal dilatation
VUJ	As above, with ureteric dilatation
PUV	As above, with distended bladder; +/– oligohydramnios
Cystic dysplasia	Small, bright, featureless; cysts; +/– oligohydramnios
MCDK	Varying size, non-communicating cysts; no parenchyma
ARPKD	Large, bright, featureless; +/– oligohydramnios
ADPKD	Large, bright; may not see discrete cysts antenatally
Malformation syndromes:	
Bardet–Biedl syndrome	Polydactyly
Meckel-Gruber syndrome	Syndactyly; posterior fossa brain abnormality

ADPKD: autosomal dominant polycystic kidney disease; ARPKD: autosomal recessive polycystic kidney disease; MCDK: multicystic dysplastic kidneys; PUJ: pelviureteric junction, PUV: posterior urethral valve; VUJ:vesicouretic junction.

40–50% of post-natal scans will be normal. Severe (>15 mm) RPD, particularly if progressive and associated with intrarenal calyceal dilatation (Fig. 8.2), is suggestive of obstruction, either pelviureteric junction obstruction, or vesicoureteric junction obstruction if the ureter is also dilated. A Tc-99 MAG-3 (mercaptoacetyltriglycine) renogram will support the diagnosis of obstruction when there is poor drainage, and impaired function on the hydronephrotic side. Surgery (pyeloplasty or ureteric reimplantation) is likely in these cases.

The main area of debate lies in the investigation of infants with mild to moderate (5–15mm) non-progressive RPD. Common practice includes use of prophylactic trimethoprim for at least the first year, and clinical follow-up with ultrasound monitoring of RPD, but not MCUG (micturating cysto-urethrogram); or an early MCUG and then prophylactic trimethoprim only for infants with proven VUR (vesico-ureteric reflux). In those infants who do have proven VUR, there is variation in practice over subsequent investigations.

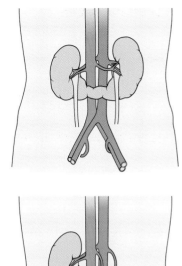
(a)

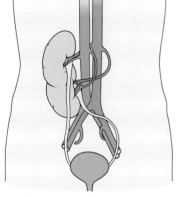
(b)

Figure 8.1 Congenital urological abnormalities. (a) Horseshoe kidney. (b) Renal ectopia. Adapted from *Urology*, with permission from Blackwell Publishing Ltd.

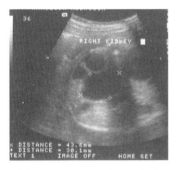

Figure 8.2 Antenatal ultrasound scan showing marked renal pelvic and calyceal dilatation.

Table 8.2 Presentation of urinary tract infections in children

Age group	Most common symptoms	→		Least common symptoms
Neonates	Fever, vomiting, lethargy, irritability	Poor feeding, failure to thrive		Abdominal pain, jaundice, haematuria, offensive urine
Pre-verbal children	Fever	Abdominal pain or abdominal/loin tenderness, vomiting, poor feeding		Lethargy, irritability, haematuria, offensive urine, failure to thrive
Verbal children	Frequent dysuria	Dysfunctional voiding, changes to continence, abdominal pain or tenderness		Fever, malaise, vomiting, haematuria, offensive urine, cloudy urine

Any child can present with septic shock secondary to urinary tract infection (UTI), although this is more common in infants. Fever is defined as >38°C. Children presenting with a UTI need a two week course of antibiotics and may need referral for imaging to rule out structural abnormalities.

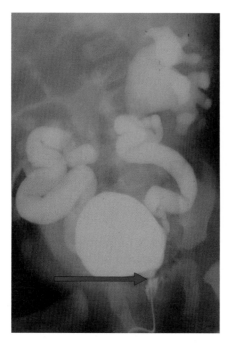

Figure 8.3 Micturating cysto-urethrogram (MCUG) showing filling defect in urethra (PUV) and gross bilateral reflux with dilatation of collecting systems.

Posterior urethral valve (PUV)

PUV is an important cause of renal failure in male infants and boys. Antenatal RPD is usually bilateral, and associated with ureteric dilatation and a persistently distended bladder. In more severe cases there is cystic change in the renal parenchyma and oligohydramnios, which may lead to pulmonary hypoplasia and life-threatening respiratory failure at delivery. MCUG is essential in this clinical setting (Fig. 8.3). Meticulous follow-up with combined nephrological and urological care is required. Dialysis and transplantation, and bladder augmentation surgery, may be needed.

Dysplastic kidneys

These are the commonest cause of chronic renal failure overall in infancy and childhood. Antenatal appearances include echobright, featureless, and often small kidneys, sometimes with identifiable cysts (Fig. 8.4). Oligohydramnios is a sign predicting poor renal function.

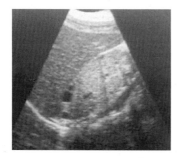

Figure 8.4 Bright featureless dysplastic kidney containing cysts.

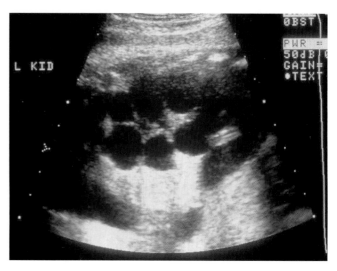

Figure 8.5 Antenatal ultrasound scan showing multiple cysts and absent parenchyma – multicystic dysplastic kidneys (MCDK).

Multicystic dysplastic kidneys

Multicystic dysplastic kidneys (MCDK) are usually diagnosed on antenatal scans, and may mimic severe hydronephrosis. There are irregular cysts of variable size from small to several centimetres, and no normal parenchyma (Fig. 8.5), with no function on a MAG-3 or DMSA (dimercaptosuccinic) scan. The ureter is dysplastic and atretic. There is a 20–40% incidence of VUR into the contralateral normal kidney, though if that kidney is normal on ultrasound, there is no indication to perform a MCUG. Current practice is not to remove the MCDK unless it is large, increasing in size, and causing pressure symptoms.

Duplex kidneys

These are usually detected when one or both moieties are dilated. The commonest abnormalities are

- obstructed hydronephrotic upper moiety and ureter, often poorly functioning and dysplastic, associated with bladder ureterocoele;
- ectopically inserted upper pole ureter, entering the urethra or vagina; this may cause true continual incontinence with no dry periods at all;
- VUR into lower pole ureter, causing infection and scarring of this pole (Fig. 8.6).

Polycystic kidney disease

Polycystic kidney disease in infancy and childhood may be autosomal recessive or dominant. Autosomal recessive polycystic kidney disease (ARPKD) has various clinical presentations, including:

- large echobright kidneys with loss of corticomedullary differentiation on antenatal ultrasound (Fig. 8.7);
- large palpable renal masses and respiratory distress at birth or early infancy;
- signs and symptoms of chronic renal failure and hypertension at any time.

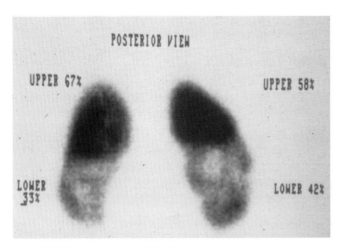

Figure 8.6 Dimercaptosuccinic (DMSA) scan of bilateral duplex kidneys with scarring of both lower moieties.

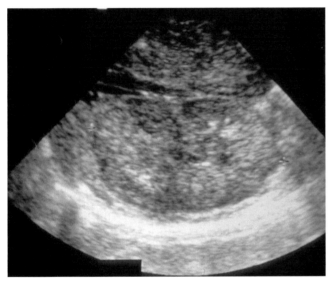

Figure 8.7 Ultrasound showing autosomal recessive polycystic kidney.

The median age for onset of established renal failure (ERF) is around 12 years, though it may cause severe renal failure in infancy; there is very variable disease severity even within same family. ARPKD is always associated with congenital hepatic fibrosis, which may vary from a subclinical association, to causing liver disease as the dominant clinical feature; complications include ascending cholangitis and portal hypertension.

Inherited, tubular and metabolic diseases

In addition to polycystic kidney disease (above), a number of other genetically-determined conditions may present during childhood. The molecular genetic basis is being identified for an increasing number of these conditions.

Alport's syndrome

This is hereditary nephritis with sensorineural deafness and coni-cal deformity of the lens of the eye. It is usually X-linked. Female carriers all have microscopic haematuria, and up to 15% may show some renal impairment in late adult life. It usually presents with an incidental finding of microscopic haematuria, or an episode of macroscopic haematuria. Deafness is first noted around 10 years, hypertension in the mid-teens, and it progresses to ERF at an average age of 21 years.

Nephronophthisis

This is an autosomal recessive condition, and the most common genetic cause of ERF in the first two decades of life. Patients have polyuria from a concentrating defect, giving a history of enuresis and bed-wetting, growth delay, often severe anaemia, and a typically 'bland' urinalysis. When associated with tapeto-retinal degeneration, it is known as Senior–Löken syndrome.

Bartter's syndrome

This is caused by an autosomal recessive defect leading to profound salt and water wasting. Symptoms are polyuria, polydipsia, episodes of dehydration, failure to thrive, and constipation; there may be maternal polyhydramnios. The characteristic biochemical disturbance is hypochloraemic hypokalaemic alkalosis, with inappropriately high levels of urinary Cl^- and Na^+.

Fanconi's syndrome

This is characterized by diffuse proximal tubular dysfunction, leading to excess urinary loss of:
- glucose: glycosuria with normal blood glucose;
- phosphate: hypophosphataemic rickets;
- bicarbonate: leading to proximal renal tubular acidosis;
- potassium: causing hypokalaemia;
- sodium, chloride and water: leading to polyuria and polydipsia, chronic extracellular fluid (ECF) volume depletion, failure to thrive, and craving for salty foods, e.g. Marmite;
- amino acids: no obvious clinical consequence.

The main causes are rare conditions, including cystinosis, tyrosinaemia, Lowe's syndrome (oculo-cerebro-renal syndrome), galactosaemia, Wilson's disease, and heavy metal toxicity (lead; mercury; cadmium).

X-linked hypophosphataemic rickets

This is also known as Vitamin D resistant rickets, and results in phosphate wasting, hypophosphataemia, delayed growth, and rickets. Treatment includes Vitamin D analogues (calcitriol or alfacalcidol), and phosphate supplements. Therapy may be complicated by hypercalcaemia and nephrocalcinosis.

Primary hyperoxaluria

This is an autosomal recessive disorder characterized by an enzyme defect leading to excess hepatic oxalate production and increased urinary excretion, with eventual calcium oxalate precipitation in the kidneys, leading to nephrocalcinosis and renal failure. Therapeutic strategies include isolated liver transplantation, if renal failure has not developed, or combined liver and kidney transplantation.

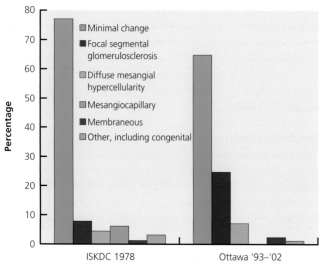

Major published series of cases of nephrotic syndrome in children

Figure 8.8 Changing proportions of children with idiopathic nephrotic syndrome. ISKDC: International Study of Kidney Disease in Children. (Reproduced from Filler G *et al.*, *American Journey of Kidney Diseases*; **42** (6): 1107–13, 2003.)

Idiopathic childhood nephrotic syndrome

Symptoms of adult nephrotic syndrome have been covered in Chapter 4. The incidence of childhood nephrotic syndrome was traditionally quoted as approximately 1 in 50 000 children, until recent information from the US and elsewhere suggested an increasing incidence (Fig. 8.8). Children with steroid-sensitive nephrotic syndrome (80–85% of cases) have a generally good prognosis, although frequently relapsing and steroid-dependent children will need adjunctive treatment. Six months, rather than the conventional course of two months of prednisolone, has been shown to reduce the subsequent frequency of relapse. Alkylating agents, predominantly cyclophosphamide, will induce long-term remissions of up to two years in 50% of children. Levamisole may be useful in a small number of children, and ciclosporin will consistently induce remission, although with the possibility of chronic nephrotoxicity and other adverse events. Mycophenolate mofetil looks to be a promising agent.

Steroid-resistant nephrotic syndrome, usually focal segmental glomerulosclerosis on biopsy, may respond very well to ciclosporin. Unfortunately, recurrent nephrotic syndrome post-transplant occurs in up to 50%, with loss of the graft unless response is seen to intensive immunosuppression with ciclosporin, MMF and plasma exchange.

Glomerulonephritis in children

The commonest form of acute glomerulonephritis (GN) in children is post-streptococcal GN (Box 8.1). With an incidence of chronic renal failure of 2–5%, mostly in the fulminating cases, it is not always totally benign.

Henoch–Schönlein nephritis occurs in 15–62% of children with Henoch–Schönlein purpura (HSP). The majority have a mild, self-limiting course. The risk of progression to ERF is about 3% of unse-

Box 8.1 Glomerulonephritis in children

- Post-streptococcal
- Henoch–Schönlein purpura (HSP)
- Haemolytic uraemic syndrome (HUS)
- IgA nephropathy
- Mesangiocapillary glomerulonephritis
- Vasculitidies, e.g.:
  - Systemic lupus erythematosus (SLE);
  - Anti-neutrophil cytoplasmic antibodies (ANCA) positive vasculitis.
- Alport's syndrome
- Membranous nephropathy
- Thin basement membrane disease

lected HSP patients, but 25% of those with a severe initial presentation develop renal failure by age 10 years. The outcome in children with IgA nephropathy is similar to that in adults, with about 15% progressing to ERF.

Chronic vasculitides are occasionally seen, with 10–17% of lupus patients presenting under the age of 16, of whom 50–80% have renal involvement. Children tend to have more severe organ involvement, with a higher mortality (10–20% by age 10 years), and a highly variable 5-year kidney survival rate of 44–93%.

Haemolytic uraemic syndrome (HUS) remains the commonest cause (45%) of acute renal failure in childhood. It is usually associated with *E. coli* 0157:H7 enterocolitis, causing severe bloody diarrhoea progressing to acute renal failure and microangiopathic anaemia and thrombocytopenia. The incidence of pneumococcal HUS is increasing in the UK, Europe and North America. Atypical HUS is exceedingly rare.

Chronic renal failure

Inherited or congenital conditions account for 50–60% of CKD and ERF in children. Autosomal recessive diseases are more than twice as common as the cause of ERF in South Asians compared to the white population (Figs 8.9 and 8.10), and these families require greater input from all aspects of a multi-disciplinary service. The aim of management of childhood CKD is to minimize the effects on growth and development, to enable normal (or as near normal as possible) social integration and schooling, and to plan for pre-emptive transplantation if appropriate and possible. Key aspects of management of CKD include:
- intensive nutritional support, often with nasogastric or gastrostomy tube feeding;
- recognition of the need for sodium chloride, sodium bicarbonate, and extra fluid supplementation in polyuric dysplastic renal disease (a common cause of CRF);
- management of renal osteodystrophy with dietary phosphate restriction, phosphate binders (usually calcium carbonate) and vitamin D analogues (alfacalcidol);
- use of recombinant human erythropoietin in advanced CRF, to treat anaemia;

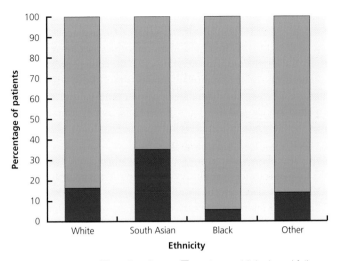

Figure 8.9 Recessive ■ vs other diseases □ causing established renal failure (ERF) by ethnicity. (Renal Registry Data 2006.)

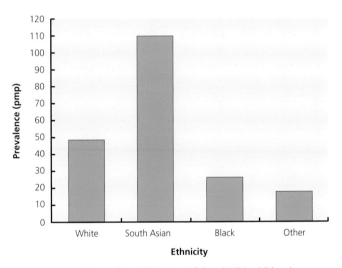

Figure 8.10 Prevalence of established renal failure (ERF) in children by ethnicity. (Renal Registry Data 2006.)

- use of recombinant human growth hormone in carefully selected patients.

Infants and children with CRF are often managed by a special clinic with input from a range of professionals including nephrologists, nurse specialists, dieticians, and pharmacists.

Renal replacement therapy

In the UK, the annual average take-on rate for RRT in children < 16 years of age is 7.7/million age-adjusted population, equating to around 100 patients per year. There are only 13 regional paediatric nephrology centres in the UK, including one each in Northern Ireland, Wales and Scotland, of which 10 provide transplantation facilities. Dialysis is possible from birth, although with routine antenatal screening and improved management of labour, it is rarely required

Table 8.3 Disadvantages of dialysis modalities

Haemodialysis	Peritoneal
Small vessels, difficult to maintain vascular access	Infection risks, especially infants in nappies or with gastrostomies
Infection risks with long-term tunnelled catheters	May not function if previous abdominal surgery
A-V fistulas associated with impaired arm growth	Parental burnout
Needle phobias and 'wriggly' small children	
>3 kg Infants	
Hospital based	
Difficult to maintain education and social interaction	

so early. Peritoneal dialysis is more practical in very small infants, but is highly stressful for families, with a high rate of 'burnout' (Table 8.3). Dialysis in children is almost always undertaken as an interim treatment with transplantation as the aim. Haemodialysis is always hospital-based, because of the difficulties maintaining vascular access in small children and their inherent cardiovascular instability. Peritoneal dialysis is usually the modality of choice (Fig. 8.11). Care of these children burdens their families with an enormous amount of travelling and disruption to normal family life, with a high rate of marital breakdown and problems with the siblings who frequently feel ignored and neglected.

Transplantation offers the best quality of life, but although graft survival rates in children of all ages are now comparable to adults (Table 8.4), re-grafting is probably inevitable at some point in the patients' lives. It is thus even more essential to strive towards improved dialysis management and better short- and long-term graft survival in this vulnerable population if we are not merely going to offer adult services to highly sensitized patients with poor dialysis access and little hope of re-transplantion. Most centres now aim pre-emptively to transplant children in order to avoid dialysis wherever possible, unless

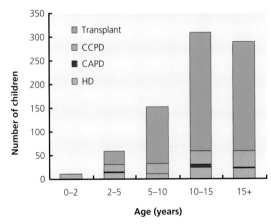

Figure 8.11 Mode of renal replacement therapy with increasing age. CAPD: continuous ambulatory peritoneal dialysis; CCPD: continuous cycling peritoneal dialysis; HD: haemodialysis. (Renal Registry Data 2005.)

Table 8.4 Figures from the National Transplant Database for paediatric recipients of first deceased donor and live donor grafts are shown, with comparable adult figures in brackets.

		Number of transplants	Survival estimate (%)
First deceased donor transplants			
One-year survival	Transplant	387 (4991)	90 (88)
	Patient	387 (4991)	99 (95)
Five-year survival	Transplant	434 (5536)	72 (72)
	Patient	434 (5536)	95 (85)
Live donor transplants			
One-year survival	Transplant	189 (1582)	94 (94)
	Patient*	173 (1386)	97 (98)
Five-year survival	Transplant	116 (876)	87 (84)
	Patient*	107 (759)	97 (95)

Survival rates for paediatric (age < 18 years) compared with adult (> 18 years) transplant patients. Cohorts for survival rate estimation: one-year survival, 1 Jan 1999–31 Dec 2003. Five-year survival, 1 Jan 1995–31 Dec 1999. *First grafts only. Re-grafts excluded from patient survival estimation.

medically contra-indicated. Paediatric patients receive some priority for deceased donor transplants, but waiting times are increasing, as in the adult sector. Children from ethnic minorities have longer waiting times and lower transplantation rates, as in the adult population. It is technically possible to transplant infants from 10 kg in weight (usually around 2 years in children with chronic renal failure), even with an adult kidney, and live donor transplants, usually from a parent, may therefore be considered even at this age. Live donor rates in a few paediatric centres are approaching 75%.

A particularly vulnerable group are the adolescents, especially at the time of transfer to adult services, when there is an unacceptably high rate of acute rejection and graft loss due to non-adherence. This is being addressed with the development of more sympathetic and effective transition procedures.

Further Reading

Rees L, Webb NJA, Brogan PA. (2007) *Paediatric Nephrology (Oxford Specialist Handbooks for Paediatrics)*. Oxford University Press, Oxford.

Webb N, Postlethwaite RJ. (eds) (2003) *Clinical Paediatric Nephrology*, 3rd edn. Oxford University Press, Oxford.

CHAPTER 9

Conservative ('Non Dialytic') Treatment for Patients with Chronic Kidney Disease

Frances Coldstream, Neil S Sheerin

OVERVIEW

- Patients need to be given information about prognosis and quality of life whether they are on dialysis, choose to stop, or even choose not to start dialysis in the first place.
- Patients with stage 4–5 CKD often have slowly progressive disease and may survive many months or even years without dialysis. However, prediction of survival can be difficult and patients can deteriorate rapidly, have a slow steady decline in function, or a decline punctuated by recurrent acute problems.
- In some patients dialysis may offer little or no significant survival rate improvement.
- There is increased recognition of a need for co-ordinated management of end-of-life care for patients with established renal failure.
- For patients who choose not to dialyse it is important to offer treatment for other aspects of CKD, for example erythropoietin therapy and phosphate control.
- Symptoms such as dry skin, itching, nausea and vomiting, constipation, anorexia, muscle cramps, abdominal bloating, insomnia and fatigue all need to be considered and treated where possible.
- Collaboration with palliative care services may be appropriate.

Introduction

As with any major organ failure severe renal disease (stage 5 CKD or ERF, GFR < 15 mL/min) is associated with significant morbidity and increased mortality. Over the last three decades, long-term renal replacement with dialysis has become increasingly available to older people and those with greater co-morbidity. However, it is now recognized that continuing or initiating dialysis may not always offer an improved quantity or quality of life; indeed, we run the risk of worsening patient outcome. In this context, palliative (also referred to as conservative, supportive or end-of-life) treatment options should be part of our management of renal failure. We need to offer realistic choices to patients with ERF but can only do so if appropriate services and support are in place.

It is important to state that this non-dialytic approach is not as a result of the chronic underfunding of renal services in the NHS. Conservative management is also seen in healthcare services where remuneration follows dialysis decisions.

Which renal patients need palliative care?

Palliative care is important for many patients with ERF. For the majority, if not all patients, end-of-life issues should be addressed prior to the introduction of renal replacement therapy. Dialysis is, after all, a treatment and not a cure. The difficulty is to decide who are most in need. Murray *et al.* (2005) suggest we ask the question, 'Would I be surprised if my patient were to die in the next 12 months?'. It then becomes clearer how many ERF patients may need input. This approach could apply to patients who choose not to have dialysis or those who would not tolerate dialysis and are treated conservatively. Patients may also choose to stop dialysis, perhaps because of the development of intercurrent illness, which may make dialysis medically impossible, or there may be an acknowledgement of a failure to tolerate, or benefit from, dialysis treatment.

The extent of the clinical need

The number of patients requiring dialysis has increased steadily, and is predicted to continue to rise for the next 20 years. Older people receiving haemodialysis will constitute a major proportion of this

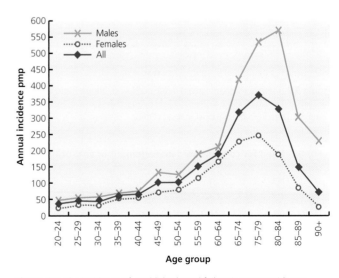

Figure 9.1 The incidence of established renal failure increases with age. Source: the Renal Registry (Ansell *et al.*, 2004).

increase due to the high incidence of renal failure in this group (Fig. 9.1) and the increasing age of the population (Fig. 9.2). The incidence of dialysis-requiring renal failure increases with age, peaking at 567 per million population (pmp) in males over 80 years. This compares with 45 pmp in men in their 20s. This may underestimate the true incidence of ERF due to unrecognized or unreferred renal failure.

The older group of patients has a high level of co-morbidity. Around 67% of patients over the age of 65 commencing dialysis have one or more significant co-morbidities that may adversely affect survival. Age and co-morbidity are strongly linked in dialysis candidates; co-morbidity is one factor that contributes to high mortality rates on dialysis, with 28% of patients over 85 years old dying in the first 90 days of starting dialysis, and this in selected patients for whom it was thought dialysis would be beneficial.

This need for co-ordinated management of end-of-life care for patients with ERF has been recognized in the *National Service Framework for Renal Services* (Box 9.1). This has both acknowledged this important phase of patient care (Fig. 9.3), and set a series of standards for the delivery of end-of-life care to patients with renal disease (Box 9.2). In addition, the UK CKD guidelines recommend referral or discussion of all people who have stage 4 or 5 CKD to nephrology services for an assessment, even if it is thought that dialysis will not be appropriate (e.g. terminal malignancy, terminal cardiac or lung disease).

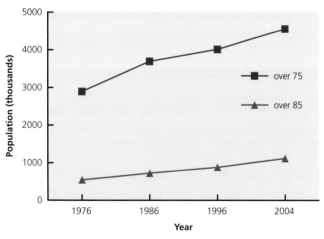

Figure 9.2 There is a steady increase in the number of people living beyond 75 years old at which stage in life established renal failure is increasingly common. Data from the National Statistics Office.

Box 9.1 Need for co-ordinated management of end-of-life care

'People with established renal failure receive timely evaluation of their prognosis, information about the choices available to them, and for those near end-of-life a jointly agreed palliative care plan, built around their individual needs and preferences.'
Source: *National Service Framework for Renal Services, Part 2* (Department of Health, 2005).

Box 9.2 Standards for the delivery of end-of-life care

'The renal multi-skilled team has access to expertise in the discussion of end-of-life issues, including those of culturally diverse groups and varied age groups, the principles of shared decision making, training in symptom relief relevant to advanced non-dialysed established renal failure (ERF).

Prognostic assessment based on available data offered to all patients with stage 4 CKD as part of the preparation for RRT.

People receive timely information about the choices available to them, such as ending RRT and commencing non-dialytic therapy, and have a jointly agreed palliative care plan built around individual needs and preferences.

People who are treated without dialysis receive continuing medical care including all appropriate non-dialytic aspects of CKD, and wherever possible are involved in decisions about medication options.

Individuals are supported to die with dignity, and their wishes met wherever practicable regarding where to die, their religious and cultural beliefs, and the presence of the people closest to them.

The care plan includes culturally appropriate bereavement support for family, partners, carers and staff.'
Source: *National Service Framework for Renal Services, Part 2* (Department of Health, 2005).

Conservative management of patients choosing not to dialyse

The decision not to dialyse can only be made after discussion between the multidisciplinary renal team and the patient, relatives and carers. The patient needs to be given information about prognosis and quality of life with or without dialysis (Fig. 9.4). Information about this is scarce. Patients with stage 4–5 CKD often have slowly progressive disease and may survive many months or even years without dialysis. If patients are assessed appropriately it is possible to identify those for whom dialysis offers little or no significant survival advantage and advise accordingly (Smith *et al.*, 2003). However, predicting survival, with or without dialysis, can be difficult. Patients can deteriorate rapidly, have a slow steady decline in function, or a decline punctuated by recurrent acute problems.

It is important that this is not seen as a 'no treatment' option, and patients are offered treatment for other aspects of CKD, for example erythropoietin therapy and phosphate control. We also need to be able actively to support these patients as end-of-life approaches.

For some patients choosing dialysis, there may be few easy treatment options. Unit-based haemodialysis will typically require patients to travel to a unit, which may be geographically distant, three times per week for dialysis treatment. The effect of treatment and its complications (e.g. infection related to dialysis access) on quality of life, particularly in elderly patients with significant co-morbidity, can be great and needs to be considered thoroughly when planning management.

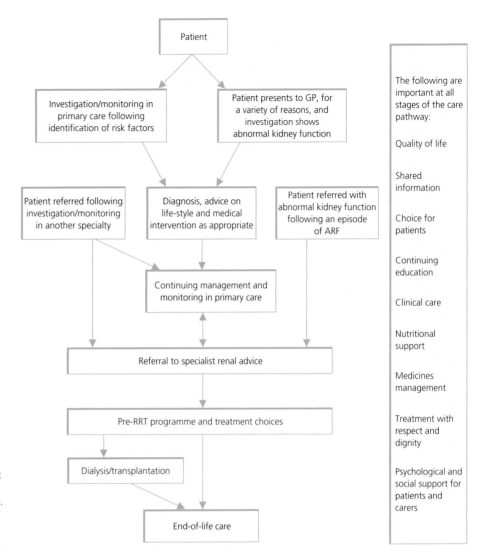

Figure 9.3 The pathway for the management of patients with renal disease recognizes that end-of-life issues are important for all patients. ARF: acute renal failure.
Source: *National Service Framework for Renal Services, Part 2* (Department of Health, 2005).

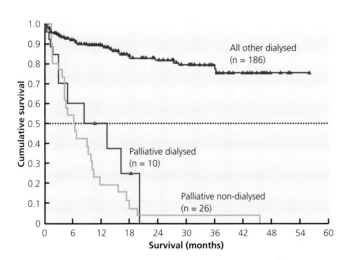

Figure 9.4 In patients who despite assessment and agreement did not elect to have dialysis, who then subsequently did have dialysis, there was not an improvement in survival. Source: Smith *et al.* (2003).

Withdrawal from dialysis

Patients may actively choose to withdraw from dialysis, or dialysis may be stopped if it is no longer providing clinical benefit. In the UK, withdrawal from dialysis is now the commonest cause of death after the first 90 days in patients over 75 years.

The prognosis after withdrawal of dialysis depends on whether the patient has residual renal function. Residual renal function is progressively lost on dialysis, particularly haemodialysis, and many dialysis patients may eventually become anuric. On stopping dialysis these patients will usually die within a few weeks. They therefore have different clinical and support needs than those choosing not to dialyse from the outset.

Symptoms: identification and control

The symptom burden related to ERF is perhaps greater than previously thought, even in those patients on renal replacement therapy (Box 9.3). Studies of symptom prevalence suggest that symptoms

Box 9.3 **Symptom burden related to ERF**

- Fatigue and lack of energy
- Itching
- Pain
- Sleep disturbance
- Restless legs
- Anxiety and/or depression
- Anorexia
- Constipation
- Cough and dyspnoea
- Nausea and vomiting

Box 9.4 **End-of-life issues**

- Symptom management
- Social support
- Psychological support
- Spiritual care
- Carer support
- Bereavement support

Table 9.1 Comparison of symptoms in established renal failure (ERF) on dialysis with other end-of-life populations

Symptom prevalence %	ERF (%)	Cancer (%)	Chronic obstructive pulmonary disease (%)	Heart disease (%)
Pain	47–50	35–96	34–77	41–77
Depression	5–60	3–77	37–71	9–36
Fatigue	73–87	32–90	68–80	69–82
Sleep disorder	31–71	9–69	55–65	36–48
Breathlessness	11–62	10–70	90–95	60–88
Anorexia	25–62	30–92	35–67	21–41
Nausea	30–43	6–68	–	17–48

Data from a systematic review of the literature by Solano *et al.* (2006) shows the minimum and maximum reported incidence of each symptom.

may be as frequent and as severe in ERF as in malignant disease or other progressive chronic diseases (Table 9.1). This is true not only in patients withdrawing from or not dialysing but also in patients actively dialysing. Symptoms such as anorexia, anxiety and depression are common to many chronic, progressive diseases whilst others such as pruritus and restless legs may be more specific to renal disease. Control of symptoms can prove difficult with the added complexity of altered drug excretion in ERF.

Anaemia, so common in CKD stages 4 and 5, can easily be treated by iron and, where needed, erythropoietin therapy (see Appendix 2). Breathlessness can be ameliorated by oxygen, by treatment of acidosis by oral sodium bicarbonate, of fluid overload by diuretics, and anaemia as above. Clonazepam can be useful in restlessness while gabapentin can help uraemic pruritus and neuropathy (but needs to be used sparingly as it can accumulate). Pain relief can be effected by trans-cutaneous patches, e.g. fentanyl, rather than primary use of oral opiates, which accumulate significantly in renal failure.

Unless specifically asked, patients will often under-report symptoms. A systematic approach, perhaps based on symptom questionnaires, may therefore be useful. Patients with ERF may also have symptoms due to co-morbid conditions that may require specific intervention.

Advanced planning

With patients who choose not to dialyse or for patients who express a wish to withdraw from dialysis, early advance planning is key. This

should include discussing what treatment a patient would want during an acute deterioration in health, describing what resuscitation means, and whether an ITU admission should take place. In addition, discussion about preferred place of care (including preferred place of death) should be included. Some patients may want to formalize their wishes by writing them down. It is likely that advanced directives will be increasingly used in this context. The healthcare team need accurately to document and communicate the patient's wishes to all individuals involved in the patient's care. It is essential to ensure that these decisions and plans are regularly revisited to ensure they are still in line with the wishes of the patient and that the appropriate care options are in place.

Links with palliative care services

Palliative care for non-cancer diseases is a rapidly developing area. As with other organ failure, there are both generic and disease-specific considerations for the treatment of patients with ERF. There needs to be close collaboration between existing renal and palliative services, both community and hospital-based, to develop management pathways for ERF patients.

Conclusions

Patients will start under the care of renal services and as their disease progresses and their end-of-life approaches they will need increasing palliative input. This change needs to be as seamless as possible. It may include a long period during which both services are involved in the care of an individual patient, as well as an extended multidisciplinary group including general practitioners, nursing services, occupational and physiotherapists, counsellors and chaplains (Box 9.4).

Further reading

Addington-Hall JM, Higginson IJ. (eds) (2001) *Palliative Care Needs for Non Cancer Patients*. Oxford University Press, Oxford.

Ansell D, Feest T, Ahmed A, Rao R. (2004) *The Seventh Annual Report*. UK Renal Registry. Available online at URL http://www.renalreg.com/Report%202004/Cover_Frame.htm

Chambers EJ, Germain M, Brown E. (eds) (2004) *Supportive Care for the Renal Patient*. Oxford University Press, Oxford.

Cohen LM, Germain M, Poppel DM, Woods A, Kjellstrand CM. (2000) Dialysis discontinuation and palliative care. *American Journal of Kidney Diseases*; **36** (**1**): 140–4.

Davison SN. (2005) Chronic pain in end-stage renal disease. *Advances in Chronic Kidney Disease*; **12** (3): 326–34.

Department of Health (2004) *National Service Framework for Renal Services. Part 1 Dialysis and Transplantation*. HMSO, London.

Department of Health (2005) *National Service Framework for Renal Services. Part 2.* HMSO, London.

Holley JL. (2005) Palliative care in end-stage renal disease: focus on advance care planning, hospice referral, and bereavement. *Seminars in Dialysis*; **18** (2): 154–6.

Murray SA, Boyd K, Sheikh A. (2005) Palliative care in chronic illness. *British Medical Journal*; **330** (7492): 611–12.

Smith C, Da Silva-Gane M, Chandna S *et al.* (2003) Choosing not to dialyse: evaluation of planned non-dialytic management in a cohort of patients with end-stage renal failure. *Nephron Clinical Practice*; **95** (2): c40–c46.

Solano JP, Gomes B, Higginson IJ. (2006) A comparison of symptom prevalence in far advanced cancer, AIDS, heart disease, chronic obstructive pulmonary disease and renal disease. *Journal of Pain and Symptom Management*; **31** (1): 58–69.

CHAPTER 10

Dialysis

Christopher W McIntyre, James O Burton

OVERVIEW

- Indications to commence dialysis are:
  - intractable hyperkalaemia;
  - acidosis;
  - uraemic symptoms (nausea, pruritis, malaise);
  - therapy-resistant fluid overload;
  - CKD stage 5.
- There is considerable variation at the level of GFR individuals may tolerate before becoming markedly uraemic.
- 'Crash-landing' onto dialysis confers a reduction in patient survival that persists for at least the first three years of subsequent therapy.
- Early identification and assiduous preparation mentally and physically are needed in the pre-dialysis phase for those likely to need renal replacement therapy.
- Haemodialysis involves circulating blood through a disposable dialyser. The vascular access of choice is the arteriovenous fistula. This, however, requires suitable peripheral veins and needs four to eight weeks for the fistula to mature. If there are no suitable veins, a graft can usually be inserted. Acute access with venous catheters has a high complication rate.
- Peritoneal dialysis involves using the peritoneum as the dialysis membrane, with pre-packaged fluid being instilled into the peritoneal space via a Tenckhoff catheter. This is usually only inserted once the decision to start dialysis is made.
- Haemodialysis is usually performed in four-hour sessions, three times a week, in hospital-based dialysis units.
- Peritoneal dialysis typically involves continuous ambulatory peritoneal dialysis (CAPD), which allows continuous dialysis using three to five exchanges of fluid per day via disposable bags.
- Automated peritoneal dialysis (APD), whereby larger volumes of fluid are instilled and drained by the use of a small machine by the bedside, is used when either more intense dialysis is needed or when, for social reasons, the night is the preferred time for treatment.

Introduction

Thomas Graham described the founding principles of dialysis over 100 years ago. Even though the first treatments for acute renal failure were performed in the 1920s, chronic dialysis treatment for established renal failure did not become a reality until 1960. In the fol-

lowing few years, a series of breakthroughs in both dialysis technology and vascular access enabled chronic renal replacement therapy (RRT) to become established in both the US and Europe by the mid 1960s. Chronic haemodialysis (HD) became widely available in the UK in the early 1970s (largely as a home-based therapy), and continuous ambulatory peritoneal dialysis (CAPD) became increasingly popular during the early 1980s. There are now some 1.5 million patients receiving regular dialysis worldwide and around 25 000 in the UK alone (Box 10.1 and Figure 10.1).

Indications for starting renal replacement therapy

There is relatively little difference in opinion about intractable hyperkalaemia, acidosis, uraemic symptoms (nausea, pruritus, malaise) and therapy-resistant fluid overload being firm indications to commence dialysis. There is, however, wider variation in clinical practice as to when to start a relatively asymptomatic patient. A cut-off based on measured or calculated GFR may be applied. In general this would be set in the CKD stage 5 range (estimated GFR ~ 10–15 mL/min). The advantages of such a 'well start' are multiple, and allow for maintenance of health prior to the development of significant abnormali-

Box 10.1 **Some basic facts about renal replacement therapy (RRT) in the UK**

- The most common cause of end-stage renal disease is diabetic nephropathy.
- Demand for dialysis will continue to increase over the next 10 years by as much as 150% for haemodialysis.
- The minimum estimated prevalence of RRT in the UK at the end of 2003 was 632 patients per million population.
- Of new patients, 22% starting RRT are >75 years old and 12% of all prevalent patients are >75 years old.
- In 2003, 67.5% of RRT patients received haemodialysis and 29.2% peritoneal dialysis (3.3% had a transplant).
- The average cost of dialysis is £30 000 per patient per year.
- The cost of a kidney transplant is £20 000 per patient per transplant with immunosuppression costs of £6500 per patient per year.
- Mortality rate in dialysis patients is about 20% annually.
- Commonest cause of death is cardiovascular disease, the risk of which is 30 times higher in dialysis patients than age-matched controls.

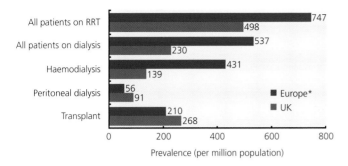

Figure 10.1 Patient numbers and modalities of treatment in established renal failure (ERF).

ties in either overall function or body composition. Furthermore, it allows dialysis provision to be built up slowly to compensate for further reduction of residual renal function (RRF). There is however still no robust (randomized controlled) evidence-base for such an approach. It is important to note that there is considerable variation in the level of GFR individuals may tolerate before becoming markedly uraemic. This may necessitate even earlier starts. The potential price for later initiation is that sudden decompensation may occur, requiring emergency treatment and a 'crash' landing onto dialysis. This confers a reduction in patient survival that persists for at least the first three years of subsequent therapy.

The general indications for starting dialysis are summarized in Table 10.1.

Preparation for renal replacement therapy

Timely and effective preparation for RRT, as well as assiduous management of the complications of CKD, is crucial. Optimal therapy whilst on dialysis will only partially compensate for previous deficiencies in care, with hypertension, functional/structural cardiovas-

cular disease, malnutrition, parathyroid hyperplasia and renal bone disease already being well established in the pre-dialysis phase. There are a number of key issues, covered below, which require a properly configured multidisciplinary team. They need to be delivered in the most effective and appropriate way for an individual's social and ethnic context.

Choice of dialysis modality

Although there may be certain overriding medical or social imperatives, the choice between PD and HD (either unit or home based) should be free, and not constrained by either clinician's prejudice or resource issues. Sufficient time and information must be provided to allow patients and families to make this choice. Poor or compelled choice will result in a higher chance of treatment failure, and poorer long-term outcomes (therapies are summarized in Table 10.2).

Dialysis access

The vascular access of choice for HD remains the arteriovenous fistula (AVF). This requires the anastomosis of an artery to a suitable segment of vein (usually either at the wrist or in the antecubital fossa). This section of vein receives arterial pressure blood and becomes 'arterialized'. This results in a structure with a thick wall, readily accessible, and with adequate flow within it to sustain an extracorporeal circuit. If there are no suitable peripheral veins, then a piece of synthetic material can be inserted (usually a PTFE graft) and this is subsequently needled for access. For the reasons of the time taken for the AVF to mature (4–8 weeks), and an initial failure rate, which may be as high as 30% (especially in older, arteriopathic or diabetic patients), this procedure must be performed in good time (Renal NSF recommends 6 months in advance of likely need). A Tenckhoff catheter for PD, to allow fluid to be instilled into the peritoneal cavity, can be inserted either at laparotomy, laparoscopically or percutaneously, but usually once the decision to start dialysis has been made (Fig. 10.2).

Dietary restriction

Specialist dietetic interaction is needed to establish the degree of restriction required in potassium, phosphate, sodium and water intake. The final diet though must maintain a reasonable level of protein intake (1 g/kg/day) and avoid malnutrition.

Treatment of anaemia

This may require correction of absolute and/or functional iron deficiency or other haematinics and starting erythropoietin therapy (see Appendix 2).

Psychosocial issues

Support for both the patient and their family is required for the psychological impact of RRT, and also practical guidance from a specialist social worker into the benefits etc. that are available if work becomes problematical. Sexual function is often affected, with problems with both libido and erectile dysfunction (amenable to the conventional range of interventions). Although fertility in women of child-bearing age is impaired, effective contraception is essential due to the immense problems associated with pregnancy whilst on dialysis. These risks are largely normalized by successful transplantation.

Table 10.1 Indications for renal replacement therapy

Acute renal failure (see Chapter 7)		CKD*	
Hyperkalaemia	K persistently >6.5. ECG changes	CKD stage 5	eGFR <15mL/min
Acidosis	pH <7.1 resistant to medical therapy	Hyperkalaemia	
Fluid overload	Particularly if compromising lung function	Fluid overload	
Symptomatic uraemia	Pericarditis Neuropathy Encephalopathy	Symptomatic uraemia	
Sepsis and multi-organ failure	Prompt intervention with RRT to prevent uraemic effects on myocardium, clotting and wound healing	Malnutrition	
Poisoning	e.g. lithium, methanol		

* Initiation of RRT in chronic renal failure varies from unit to unit. Listed are some contributing factors.
CKD: chronic kidney disease; eGFR: estimated glomerular filtration rate; RRT: renal replacement therapy.

Table 10.2 Relative advantages and disadvantages of haemo- and peritoneal dialysis

	Haemodialysis	Peritoneal dialysis
Methods and procedures	Three four-hour sessions a week, usually in hospital Some flexibility with days and sessions Not reliant on patient's ability to learn or carry out procedures	Continuous dialysis using up to four exchanges/day or cycling at night Procedure done at home and can fit more easily into lifestyle and work Reliant upon patient or other person to perform the procedure safely
Dialysis access	Acute access with venous catheters has high complication rate (infection, stenosis, thrombosis) Fistulae need 2–3 months to mature before use AV fistulae can be difficult to form in patients with vascular disease	Access relatively easy to establish Can be used immediately Comparatively more contra-indications (stoma, bowel adhesions, inoperable hernias, obesity)
Fluid balance/ ultrafiltration	Set at the beginning of dialysis and is predictable Amount of fluid to be removed is limited by cardiac function (increased risk of intradialytic hypotension)	Less predictable Controlled by concentration of dextrose (or glucose polymer) in dialysate Integrity of the peritoneum as membrane declines with time, esp. with frequent use of higher dextrose concentrations
Complications	Catheter infections and associated complications (septicaemia, SBE etc.) can be life threatening Cardiovascular death from arrhythmias, MI and stroke are increased (intradialytic hypotension predisposes)	Exit site infections are rarely serious and peritonitis, if persistent, usually resolves after removal of catheter Recurrent infections and membrane failure leads to high dropout rate Hernias and leaks from increased peritoneal pressure
Psychosocial considerations	Transport to and from the unit three times a week can disrupt patient and family schedules and prolong dialysis sessions Holidays are hard to plan as patient must rely on local dialysis facilities Body image problems associated with access/fistulae Erectile dysfunction and poor libido	Care of a family member at home can be easier Transport to hospital only needed for clinics or emergencies PD fluids can be delivered worldwide with prior notice Body image problems associated with PD catheter Erectile dysfunction and poor libido

AV: arteriovenous; PD: peritoneal dialysis; SBE: subacute bacterial endocarditis.

Renal replacement therapy

Haemodialysis

Haemodialysis involves circulating blood through a disposable dialyser. This contains hollow fibres of a selectively permeable material, giving a large total surface area (1–2 m²). Dialysate is produced by the continuous combination of concentrate with highly-treated tap water (microbiologically pure, low endotoxin concentration and depleted in minerals). This flows around the hollow fibres in the opposite direction to blood. It contains a low concentration of factors to be removed and a higher concentration of bicarbonate, allowing diffusion into the blood and correction of acidosis. Removal of accumulated fluid is achieved by applying a pressure gradient across the dialysis membrane, resulting in controlled ultrafiltration (Fig. 10.3).

Conventionally, heparin is used to prevent clotting and the treatment is performed three times a week, for 3–5 h per session. This results in adequate control of biochemistry (though not normalized), fluid overload, acidosis and uraemic symptoms in *most* patients.

Peritoneal dialysis

This technique involves using the peritoneum as the dialysis membrane. Pre-packaged fluid is instilled into the peritoneal space. It is allowed to dwell for a period of time. Waste products to be removed diffuse from the blood into the fluid. Again, the dialysate contains factors that do not need to be removed at similar concentrations to normal plasma (calcium, magnesium, sodium etc). Acidosis is corrected by the diffusion of buffer from the fluid into the blood, and ultrafiltration occurs down an oncotic gradient. This is produced by the fluid having a higher osmolality than plasma (due to a high concentration of glucose or glucose polymer within the instilled fluid).

Ready drainage relies on good tube placement and function. The most common cause of failure is constipation with tube displacement, or inspissation of omental fat into the catheter's multiple distal perforations. PD patients characteristically are prescribed aperients to ideally promote two soft bowel motions per day. The main limitations of the technique relate to the development of peritonitis, resulting from either an infected exit site, poor adherence to the technical challenges associated with PD bag changes or bacterial translocation across the bowel wall.

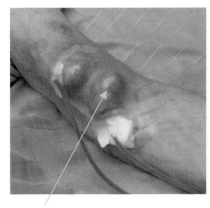

(a)　　　　　　Arterialized vein

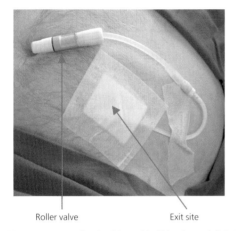

(b)　　　Roller valve　　　　　Exit site

Figure 10.2 (a) Arteriovenous fistula. (b) Tenckhoff (peritoneal dialysis, PD) catheter.

There are a number of refinements of the PD method. Continuous ambulatory PD (CAPD) involves 3–5 exchanges of fluid per day, every day (due to the intrinsically lower solute removal efficiency compared with HD). The patient performs these manually, with the bag being disconnected between each exchange.

In some patients, either more intensive dialysis is needed or for social reasons the night is the preferred time for the treatment to take place. In this setting, automated peritoneal dialysis (APD) can be used. This allows larger volumes to be instilled and drained by the use of a small machine by the bedside (Fig. 10.4).

Up until recently, the composition of all PD fluids was very similar. Glucose was used to produce the oncotic gradient and lactate was used as buffer (absorbed and converted to bicarbonate by the liver). Due to the limitations of using these compounds, and an increasing appreciation of the biological toxicities of glucose degradation products, a number of other fluids have subsequently been developed with a greater degree of biocompatibility (summarized in Table 10.3).

Monitoring adequacy of renal replacement therapy

The aim of chronic dialysis therapy is to replicate as far as possible the normal functions of the failed kidney(s). Patients are monitored, usually monthly, for a wide range of indices relating to solute clearance, mineral metabolism, volume status, nutrition and anaemia (summarized in Table 10.4).

Solute clearance
This is usually measured as small solute clearance, and the conventional marker is urea. Clearance is measured by blood sampling before

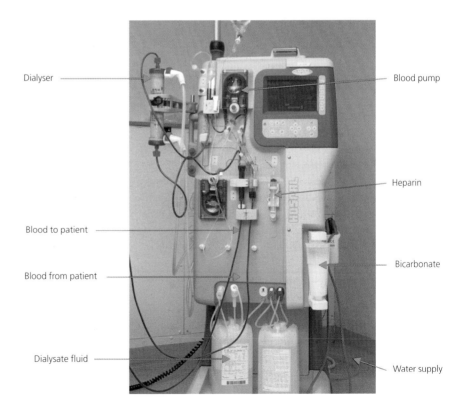

Dialyser

Blood pump

Heparin

Blood to patient

Blood from patient

Bicarbonate

Dialysate fluid

Water supply

Figure 10.3 Haemodialysis machine.

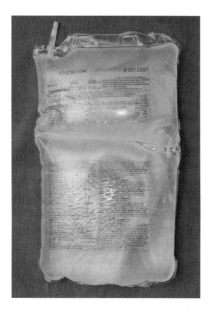

(a)

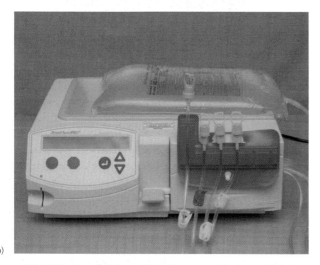

(b)

Figure 10.4 (a) Peritoneal dialysate fluid. (b) automated peritoneal dialysis (APD) machine.

and after HD, or with a combination of blood samples and samples of waste fluid in PD. A variety of mathematical treatments are applied to these measurements and the adequacy of clearance calculated. Failure to reach certain thresholds is associated with increasing symptoms, failure to thrive and increased mortality. In HD, dialyser size, blood flow through the dialyser, access quality and treatment time can all be modulated to enhance clearance. In PD the dialysate volumes, number of exchanges, dwell time and use of APD are the main factors that can be altered to vary the efficiency of dialysis. The clearance of other factors can be measured (middle molecules) and these may influence the development of some long-term complications.

Maintenance of dry/desired weight

This refers to the patient's weight best replicating the normal level of hydration (Table 10.5), and is important in managing hypertension and preventing the development of left ventricular hypertrophy and cardiac failure.

Table 10.3 Types of peritoneal dialysate fluids

Fluid type	Comments
Conventional lactate buffered glucose-based solutions	Fluid removal is dependent on glucose concentration. Low biocompatibility and high glucose degradation products.
Bicarbonate-based buffered solutions	Uses bicarbonate alone or in combination with lactate. This has been shown to reduce pain during infusion and may improve long-term preservation of the peritoneal membrane.
Glucose polymer solutions (Icodextrin)	Contains a glucose polymer less likely to be absorbed into the body. Also benefits long-term PD patients with poor ultrafiltration. It is used once each day for the long dwell. Use reduces systemic glucose exposure.
Amino acid containing solutions	Contains amino acids instead of glucose. Possibly useful for patients with malnutrition and hypoalbuminaemia. More than once daily use may result in acidosis.

Table 10.4 Treatment aims for dialysis patients

Factor	Aims
Haemoglobin	10.5–12.5 g/dL
Potassium	Haemodialysis: 3.5–6.5 mmol/L Peritoneal dialysis: 3.3–5.5 mmol/L
Calcium	Normal range
Parathyroid hormone	2–4 x normal range
Phosphate	1.2–1.7 mmol/L
Albumin	Normal range
Systolic blood pressure	≤140 mmHg pre-dialysis
Diastolic blood pressure	≤90 mmHg pre-dialysis
Adequacy	Haemodialysis: Kt/V ≥1.2 Peritoneal dialysis: Kt/V ≥1.7 (≥2.0 for APD)

APD: automated peritoneal dialysis.

Table 10.5 Monitoring fluid balance

Situation	Effects
Dehydrated	Weight loss, dizziness, nausea, constipation, hypotension, cramps
Ideal weight	Nil
Fluid overloaded	Weight increases, feet/ankles swell, breathlessness, hypertension

Anaemia

Usually requires erythropoietin therapy either subcutaneously or IV delivered during dialysis, often with IV iron supplementation (see Appendix 2).

Table 10.6 Complications of dialysis

Haemodialysis	Peritoneal dialysis
	Hypertension
	Increased cardiovascular risk
	Malnutrition
	Renal bone disease
	Anaemia
	Psychosocial/sexual factors
Intradialytic hypotension	Hernias
Adverse dialysis-related symptoms	Fluid leaks
(cramps, headache etc)	Peritonitis (+subsequent membrane/
Access issues (infection, aneurysm,	ultrafiltration failure)
thrombosis & rupture)	
Amyloid	

Residual renal function

Maintenance of RRF reduces mortality and facilitates volume management, whilst avoiding the draconian fluid restriction required in anephric patients (500–750 mL/day). NSAID usage may reduce RRF, and therefore continued caution is required even in patients established on RRT.

Mineral metabolism and renal bone disease

This requires careful modulation of phosphate binders (type and dose), vitamin D and calcimimetics/parathyroidectomy.

Other factors

These include assessment of suitability for transplantation, and monitoring of complications (Table 10.6 and Fig. 10.5).

Developments in delivery of RRT

Peritoneal dialysis continues to be an important treatment modality both in the UK and Holland – two European countries with socialized healthcare systems and chronic underfunding of haemodialysis facilities – and in particular across the developing world. Wholesale adoption of the newer and more expensive PD solutions is currently being handicapped by the lack of appropriate outcome studies, although they do seem to have a wide range of benefits in terms of peritoneal function, systemic biocompatibility and cardiovascular response.

Haemodialysis technology is also becoming more complex, with the use of biosensors to detect the physiological response to treatment and run biofeedback systems to improve treatment tolerability. Perturbations of dialysate temperature and sodium concentration, as well as adding a degree of convective clearance to dialysis, can ameliorate the common problem of intra-dialytic hypotension (IDH). These technologies, however, are largely adaptive to compensate for the high ultrafiltration rates and short treatment times driven by current pressures on dialysis resources. Increasing interest is occurring in daily dialysis (short hours during the day, or long, low efficiency treatment overnight) in either a unit or home-based environment.

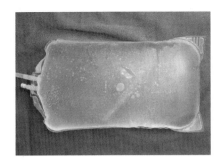

(a)

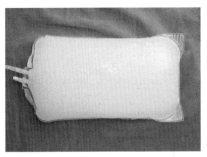

(b)

Figure 10.5 Drained fluid in peritoneal dialysis (PD) peritonitis. (a) Normal peritoneal dialysate drainage. (b) Cloudy dialysate drainage in peritonitis.

There is a resurgence of interest in home haemodialysis, with improvements in water-preparation and machine portability, and the increasing realization that with long overnight (quotidian) dialysis, or daily short-session dialysis, there can be very significant improvements in anaemia, calcium-phosphate balance, acidosis, nutrition, blood pressure, lipid profiles and left ventricular hypertrophy compared to 'standard' thrice weekly four-hour sessions.

It is certain that the escalating numbers of patients on treatment and increasing co-morbidity load will require continued refinement of RRT, whilst not replacing the need for early identification and assiduous preparation mentally and physically in the pre-dialysis phase.

Further reading

Bender FH, Bernardini J, Piraino B. (2006) Prevention of infectious complications in peritoneal dialysis: best demonstrated practices. *Kidney Int Suppl*; **70** (103): S44–54.

Greneche S, D'Andon A, Jacquelinet C et al. (2005) Choosing between peritoneal dialysis and haemodialysis: a critical appraisal of the literature. *Nephrol Ther*; **1**(4): 213–20.

Hayashi R, Huang E, Nissenson AR. (2006) Vascular access for hemodialysis. *Nat Clin Pract Nephrol*; **2**(9): 504–13.

Light P. (2006) Current understanding of optimal blood pressure goals in dialysis patients. *Curr Hypertens Rep*; **8** (5):413–9.

NHS Information National Library for Kidney Disease, www.library.nhs.uk/kidney

Rabindranath KS, Strippoli GF, Daly C et al. (2006) Haemodiafiltration, haemofiltration and haemodialysis for end-stage kidney disease. *Cochrane Database Syst Rev*; **18** (4): CD006258.

CHAPTER 11

Renal Transplantation

Ming He, John Taylor

OVERVIEW

- Kidney transplantation is generally the optimal form of renal replacement therapy in terms of patient survival, quality of life and cost-effectiveness.

- Immunosuppressive treatment is necessary for the life of the kidney transplant – hence compliance is a major issue in the graft survival.

- ABO compatibility is necessary between the donor and recipient. The risk of transplant rejection is less where there is good HLA antigen 'match'. Blood transfusions can sensitize the recipient to potential donor HLA antigens, and so should be avoided if possible when there is a likelihood of transplantation.

- A live, unrelated transplant with complete HLA mismatching has a better long-term outcome than a cadaveric organ with no mismatch at all.

- Living donors now account for 25% of all kidneys transplanted in the UK, and this is increasing.

- Post-operatively, most kidneys function immediately. Acute tubular necrosis is the single most likely cause of delayed graft function, and is usually reversible.

- The main complications of kidney transplantation are:

  - Rejection: 10–30% of transplanted kidneys are acutely rejected; this presents as a decline in renal function usually within the first three months. Hyperacute rejection, which occurs within hours, is very rare.

  - Chronic allograft nephropathy: this is the main cause of graft failure; progressive and irreversible increases in creatinine, associated with proteinuria, usually occur over years.

  - Infection: the main concern is susceptibility to opportunistic infections, notable CMV and *Pneumocystis carinii*.

  - Malignancy: increased risk of post-transplantation lymphoproliferative disorders associated with Epstein–Barr virus infection.

  - Recurrence: all forms of glomerulonephritis can recur and affect the transplanted kidney.

- Graft survival at 1 year is approximately 85–90% for cadaveric kidneys and more than 95% for living donors. Overall, graft survival is about 50% at 10 years; the main causes of graft attrition are either chronic allograft nephropathy or death of the patient.

Introduction

Kidney transplantation is the optimal form of renal replacement therapy (RRT), whether in terms of patient survival, quality of life or cost-effectiveness. However, this option is available to only about 30% of RRT patients. The number of patients on the waiting list is increasing as transplantation becomes a more established procedure (Fig. 11.1), immunosuppression regimes are refined, and previously contra-indicated recipients are also being considered (e.g. HIV positive).

As well as kidney transplantation alone, kidneys can be transplanted at the same time as a liver (e.g. cirrhosis with kidney failure, or primary hyperoxaluria), or a heart. Simultaneous kidney–pancreas transplantation is less common, but a significant treatment option for type 1 diabetic patients with established renal failure (ERF) (Fig. 11.2). Space considerations preclude more detailed descriptions.

Immunological aspects of transplantation

The almost universal need to continue immunosuppressive treatment for the life of the kidney transplant for all donor/recipient combinations means that compliance is a major issue in graft survival.

Acquired immunity consists of the cellular (T-cell mediated) and humoral (B-cell mediated) responses, and both are involved in graft rejection. Essentially, the acquired immune response depends on recognition of graft antigens as being foreign and this stimulates various effector mechanisms against the graft, such as macrophage activation, natural killer cell response, delayed hypersensitivity, cellular cytotoxicity, plus complement fixation.

Figures 11.3 and 11.4 detail the immunological barriers to transplantation, and 'matching' – the extreme polymorphism of alleles at the HLA loci mean that a degree of mismatch is likely between donor and recipient, and this is usually expressed as a mismatch score, i.e. 0–0–0 being a perfect match and 2–2–2 being a complete mismatch.

The kidney donor

There are two broad categories: cadaveric or living. Cadaveric donors are either heart-beating or non-heart-beating (NHBD). Table 11.1 shows contraindications to cadaveric kidney donation.

Cadaveric

The largest group of transplants comes from brain-stem dead patients with maintained cardiac output, usually in an ICU setting. Cause of death is usually intra-cranial haemorrhage or trauma. Kidneys from non-heart-beating donors, i.e. post-circulatory arrest, have shown

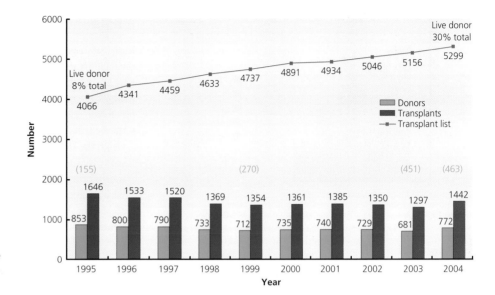

Figure 11.1 Cadaveric kidney programme in the UK, 1995–2004. Number of donors, transplants and patients on the active transplant list at 31 December each year (live donors are indicated in parentheses). Figures from United Kingdom Transplant (UKT).

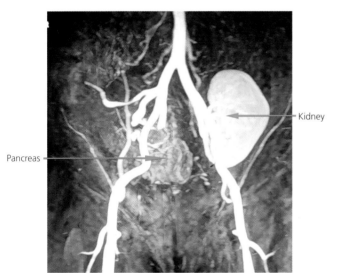

Figure 11.2 Magnetic resonance (MR) angiogram showing a kidney transplant on the right and a pancreas transplant on the left of the figure.

comparable rates of success. However, the drawback to this approach is the warm ischaemic time (the time between cessation of heartbeat with the diagnosis of death and cooling of the organ). Of all potential donors in the ITU setting, consent for donation is not forthcoming from 36% of families.

Once a donor is identified, HLA typing is carried out and the most suitable recipient found through a national matching scheme administered by the UK Transplant Support Service Authority (see website in Further reading). Clinically, peri-retrieval factors such as haemodynamic instability, ventilation, hypothermia, and diabetes insipidus are managed to optimize perfusion.

Living

This now accounts for about 25% of all kidneys transplanted in the UK (Fig. 11.1), and in some Scandinavian and American centres live transplants are more numerous than deceased donor options. Living donation is on the increase in the UK – it may become the

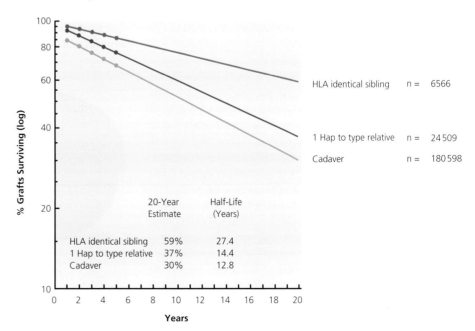

Figure 11.3 Relationship between survival and type of donor (first kidney transplants 1985–2004). (CTS-K-1503-0206)

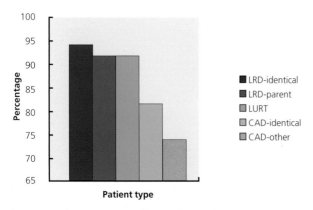

Figure 11.4 Three-year renal graft survival. UCLA data 28 945 patients. The outcome of HLA-identical cadaveric kidneys is inferior to all categories of live donor, including living unrelated transplants. CAD: cadaveric donor; LRD: living-related donor; LURD:living unrelated donor. Source: Terasaki PI *et al.* (1995) *New England Journal of Medicine;* **333**(6):333–6.

Table 11.1 Contraindications to cadaveric donation

Absolute	Relative
Chronic renal disease	Age < 5 or > 60
Potentially metastasizing malignancy	Mild hypertension
Severe hypertension	Treated infection
Bacterial septicaemia	Nonoliguric acute tubular necrosis
Current intravenous drug user	Positive hepatitis B and C serology
HIV positive	Intestinal perforation with spillage
Warm ischaemia > 45 mins	Prolonged cold ischaemia
Irreversible acute renal failure	High-risk behaviour

most practical way to address the donor organ deficit for kidneys at least, especially as live-unrelated donation (e.g. between spouses) is yielding excellent outcomes and newer surgical techniques are being employed with the benefits of reduced pain, greater cosmesis and faster post-operative recovery (e.g. laparoscopic nephrectomy). A live-unrelated transplant with complete HLA mismatching still has a better long-term outcome than a cadaveric organ with no mismatch at all (Fig. 11.3). Another advantage of living donors is the possibility of considering a 'marginal' recipient who might not be suitable for a cadaveric kidney.

The process of evaluation of the living donor is outlined fully in the Living Donor Guidelines, as set by the British Transplant Society and UK Renal Association. Patients and potential donors are given information leaflets and videos, and donors undergo a full series of screening investigations. Those who go on to donate have a risk of death of 1 in 3000, and there is no excess risk of hypertension or ERF post-donation. Regardless, monitoring of BP, urinary protein excretion and renal function in the longer term in kidney donors is important. However, the final donation rate may be as low as 20–25% in all those who are assessed as a potential live donor. The reasons for this vary from immunological (40%) and medical (20%), to donor withdrawal or uncertainty (up to 40%). All potential living donors (whether related or unrelated) are assessed independently at a local level to determine their suitability for donation under terms set out by the Human Tissue Act 2004. More complex cases can be referred to the Human Tissue Authority.

Recipient

Kidney transplantation is considered suitable for patients with chronic renal failure requiring dialysis or predicted to require dialysis within 6 to 12 months. In the UK, around 25% of such patients are transplanted, the main constraint being donor supply. The main principles to consider during recipient selection are:

* the benefits in terms of quality and duration of life should outweigh the risks to the patient in terms of the procedure and subsequent immunosuppression, especially in patients with other co-morbidities or older patients;
* with cadaveric organs, justifying the use of a limited resource and allocation should be in terms of maximum benefit to society (patients not likely to survive five years or less should not receive a cadaveric donor kidney);
* in living donors, the risk to the donor should be justified by the predicted benefit of a successful transplant.

Apart from these general issues and those pertaining to the undertaking of major surgical intervention in the context of renal disease, various specific clinical factors must be considered.

Infection

Active infections should be eradicated where possible (e.g. TB); patients with chronic hepatitis B or C can prove challenging, as post-transplantation exacerbation of virally-driven liver pathology is well recognized. Patients with recurrent urinary tract infection are considered for native nephrectomy. Those at risk of post-transplant tuberculosis should have TB prophylaxis post-operatively.

Malignancy

Patients with current malignancy are not considered for transplantation, but treated patients may be transplanted after a recurrence-free period, depending on type of malignancy.

Cardiovascular disease

As this is the most common cause of death (and hence graft loss) post-transplant (Fig. 11.5), any history or evidence of disease is thoroughly investigated and treated as appropriate. In addition certain groups of asymptomatic patients, such as those over 50 years, smokers, and all diabetics, should undergo cardiovascular screening

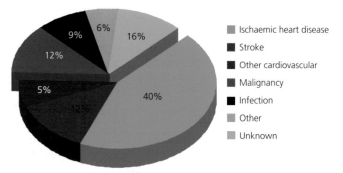

Figure 11.5 Cardiovascular disease is the major cause of death with a functioning graft in renal transplant recipients. First grafts 1984–1996 / 92 deaths in 1260 patients. Source: Kavanagh D *et al.* (1999) *Nephron;* 81(1): 109–10.

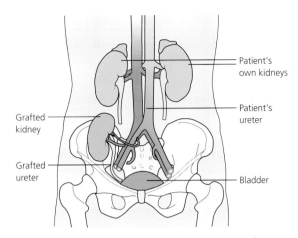

Figure 11.6 Grafted kidney placed heterotopically in the iliac fossa.

(e.g. stress echocardiography, nuclear scintigraphy, coronary angiography, iliac arterial imaging).

Bladder function

Urological problems (e.g. outflow obstruction) should be investigated before transplantation.

Surgical aspects

Donor/retrieval

Cadaveric kidneys usually come from multi-organ retrievals and are shipped on ice. The timing of the recipient transplant is set to minimize the cold ischaemic time. The shorter this is, the more likely the immediate function of the kidney – which has a positive effect on graft outcome.

Living donors can be operated on electively – for instance, timed to 'pre-empt' the need for dialysis.

Recipient

The graft is usually placed heterotopically in the iliac fossa (Fig. 11.6), which is extra-peritoneal in adults but is placed intra-peritoneally in a child weighing less than 20 kg. The iliac vessels are used in the former case and the aorta/inferior vena cava in the latter. The ureter is implanted onto the dome of the bladder. In the pelvis, the kidney is safe and there are no restrictions on recipient activity.

Post-operative management

Most kidneys function immediately – certainly those from living donors almost without fail. Immediate post-operative concerns are with fluid balance and risk of bleeding.

Deterioration in kidney function may be reversible (hypovolaemia, acute tubular necrosis, ureteric obstruction, drug toxicity especially calcineurin inhibitors, acute rejection) or irreversible (hyperacute rejection, vascular thrombosis). Ultrasound with Doppler assessment of blood flow and percutaneous biopsy should help identify these causes (Fig. 11.7).

Acute tubular necrosis is the single most likely cause of delayed graft function and tends to occur in cadaveric kidneys, especially

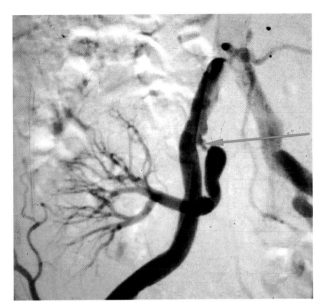

Figure 11.7 Renal transplant angiogram showing a 95% stenosis in the transplant artery (see arrow)

those from older donors and kidneys with a prolonged cold ischaemic time or from NHBD. Dialysis is required until the ATN resolves.

Immunosuppression

Immunosuppression is initiated at the time of transplant. There are various classes of immunosuppressive agents (Table 11.2), used in combination to prevent rejection and minimize dose-related side-effects (Table 11.3 and Fig. 11.8). Different agents may also be used during different phases of immunosuppressive therapy, namely induction, maintenance, and treatment of rejection episodes.

Complications

These may be complications related to surgery (as discussed briefly above), or longer-term problems related to rejection, infection, malignancy, and recurrence of the original disease – all of which have an impact on the overall outcome or success of the procedure. There is also a risk of mortality especially during the first 100 post-operative days (Fig. 11.9).

Rejection

Hyperacute rejection occurs within hours and is extremely rare. It results from the presence of pre-existing antibodies in the recipient to donor antigens. There is no effective treatment and the graft must be removed. Prevention depends on ABO matching and pre-transplant lymphocyte cross-matching.

Acute rejection occurs in 10–30% of recipients with current immunosuppressive protocols, and presents as an early decline in renal function e.g. within the first three months. It is confirmed by percutaneous needle renal biopsy and treated with high-dose steroids and some modification of the maintenance immunosuppressive regimen.

Table 11.2 Classes of immunosuppressive drugs

Corticosteroids	Broad anti-inflammatory and immunosuppresive effects; inhibit activation of T-cells. Started at transplantation with weaning off after a few months as there are numerous long-term side-effects.
Antiproliferative agents (e.g. azathioprine, mycophenolate mofetil)	Inhibits purine metabolism and DNA synthesis. Used in suppressing rejection, MMF more potent.
Calcineurin inhibitors (e.g. ciclosporin, tacrolimus)	Block the intracellular signalling pathway leading to IL-2 release and amplication of immune response. Narrow therapeutic index, requires regular blood level monitoring. Tacrolimus is more potent.
Cell cycle inhibitors (e.g. sirolimus)	Prevents proliferation of T-cells, more potent than ciclosporin but not nephrotoxic. Reduces the incidence of acute rejection.
Biological agents (e.g. OKT3, basiliximab, daclizimab, ALG, ATG)	Monoclonal antibodies targeting CD3 or the IL-2 receptor have a role in the treatment of acute rejection. They are associated with cytokine release syndrome. IL-2 receptor antagonist given at induction reduces acute rejection.

Table 11.3 Principal side-effects of immunosuppressive therapy

Corticosteroids	Ciclosporin	Tacrolimus	Azathioprine	Mycophenolate mofetil	Sirolimus
Hypertension	Nephrotoxic effects	Nephrotoxic effects	Marrow suppression	Diarrhoea/gastrointestinal upset	Dyslipidaemia
Glucose intolerance	Hypertension	Hypertension		Marrow suppression	Marrow suppression
Dyslipidaemia	Glucose intolerance	Glucose intolerance			Acne
Osteoporosis	Dyslipidaemia	Dyslipidaemia			Poor wound healing
	Gum hyperplasia	Alopecia			
	Hirsutism				

Modified from Denton MD *et al.* (1999) *Lancet*; **353**: 1083–91.

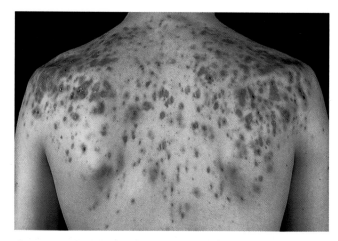

Figure 11.8 Severe acne due to steroids.

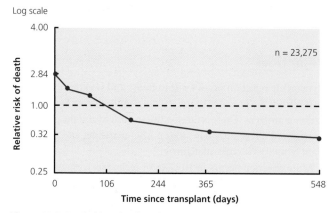

Figure 11.9 Survival benefit of renal transplantation (adapted from Wolfe RA *et al.* (1999) *New Engandl Journal of Medicine*; **341** (23): 1725–30).

Due to the need for significant and sustained surveillance of renal transplant patients (regular renal function testing), we generally recommend waiting for a clear 12 months post-transplantation period to have elapsed before sanctioning pregnancy or extended foreign travel.

Late acute rejection is a feature of poor compliance.

Chronic allograft nephropathy

This is the main cause of graft failure. Both immunological (incidence of acute rejection, degree of HLA mismatch) and non-immunological factors (hypertension, diabetes mellitus, hyperlipidaemia and chronic exposure to calcineurin inhibitors) are involved. A progressive, irreversible increase in creatinine levels is seen, particularly when associated with proteinuria. Figure 11.10 shows histopathological changes associated with chronic allograft nephropathy (CAN).

Infection

In the immediate post-operative period, bacterial infections can complicate recovery as in any surgical procedure (e.g. wound, chest, urinary tract). However, the main concern with transplant recipients is the susceptibility to opportunistic infections due to immunosuppressive therapy (Figs 11.11 and 11.12).

Cytomegalovirus is a particular concern in a seropositive to -negative transplant (Fig. 11.13), and these recipients should have routine oral prophylaxis with valganciclovir for 90 days. An alternative may be regular screening of blood for CMV DNA by PCR techniques. Viral infections may also be involved in malignancies.

Post engraftment, prophylaxis with co-trimoxazole for *Pneumocystis carinii* is given for 3 months. High-risk patients can receive isoniazid and pyroxidine for TB prophylaxis for six months.

Figure 11.10 Histology of chronic allograft nephropathy (CAN) – extracellular matrix deposition. (a) Intimal hyperplasia. (b) Interstitial fibrosis. (c) Glomerulosclerosis.

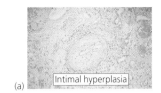 (a)
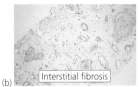 (b)
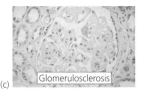 (c)

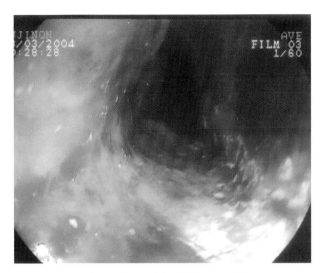

Figure 11.11 Oesophageal ulcer and slough due to candida.

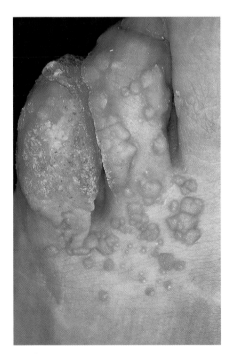

Figure 11.12 Viral warts.

Malignancy

There is a significantly increased risk for lymphoproliferative disorders post-transplantation (PTLD), which is associated with Epstein–Barr virus infection. Treatment of PTLD involves careful reduction or withdrawal of immunosuppression and starting chemotherapy regimes as appropriate.

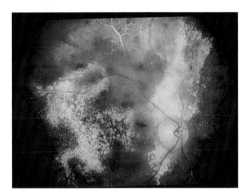

Figure 11.13 Retinal cytomegalovirus infection.

Skin malignancies, such as squamous cell carcinoma, Kaposi's sarcoma and others with a viral aetiology (e.g. human papilloma virus-related) are also much increased (Fig. 11.14).

Recurrence

All forms of glomerulonephritis (IgA nephropathy, familial haemolytic-uraemic syndrome), and some metabolic or systemic diseases (e.g. diabetes, amyloidosis) can recur after transplantation; despite this, the contribution of this cause of total loss of allograft function is small. In some unlucky individuals, disease recurrence is a feature of successive transplants. It is rarely possible to effectively treat post-transplantation disease recurrence.

Outcome

Graft survival at 1 year is approximately 85 to 90% for cadaveric kidneys and more than 95% for living donors. The attrition rate continues at a steady 3 to 5% per year (Fig. 11.15), so graft survival is about 50% at 10 years overall – hence many patients return to dialysis after 10 years or have a repeat transplant. The main causes of graft attri-

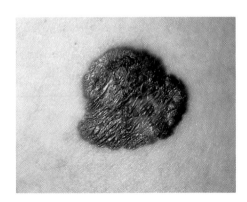

Figure 11.14 Malignant melanoma.

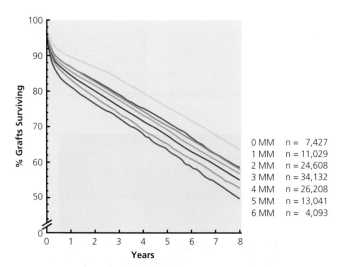

Figure 11.15 HLA-A+B+DR Mismatches (first cadaver kidney transplants 1985–2004). (CTS-K-21101-0206)

tion are chronic allograft nephropathy (CAN) and death (usually from cardiac problems). Improvements in graft survival will probably depend on an improved understanding of CAN and directed therapies to prevent it, and accurate identification and treatment of those patients with significant cardiac co-morbidity.

Living donation is associated with better graft and patient outcomes in general. It also makes pre-emptive renal transplantation more feasible, which is associated with better outcomes.

Compliance

Graft survival inevitably depends on compliance with immunosuppressive regimens, and noncompliance is a major risk factor in both acute rejection and chronic allograft nephropathy. Patients with a history of psychosocial problems such as drug addiction should be fully assessed and rehabilitated before being entered onto the transplant waiting list.

The future

There are a number of strategies to increase the quantity of organs available for donation in the near future; one of the most feasible is to increase living donation. Widening patient and public awareness from the level of the clinician to national educational campaigns

could help with this. More specifically, new legislation (Human Tissue Act, 2004) that came onto the statute book in September 2006 now permits altruistic donation, and 'organ-swapping' within two or more donor–patient pairs who had greater reciprocal HLA matching, i.e. paired or pooled donation.

Major advances using anti CD 20 antibody plasmapheresis or immunoabsorption now permit successful kidney transplantation even across some ABO blood group compatibilities and in the presence of anti HLA antibodies (i.e. sensitized patients).

Many of the current immunologically active pharmaceutical agents are imprecise and difficult to use. There is much excitement about, and anticipation of, the new generation of more precisely-targeted immunological tolerance-permitting drugs, which may be permissive of long-term accommodation, reducing the need for long-term use of potentially nephro- and cardiotoxic medications such as steroids or calcineurin inhibitors.

Xenotransplantation has been considered since the last decade but is not a practicable option at present – not least due to immune incompatibility. It is, and will always remain, the future of transplantation.

Further reading

British Transplantation Society/The Renal Association. *United Kingdom Guidelines for Living Donor Kidney Transplantation*. Available at URL http://www.bts.org.uk

EBPG Expert Group on Renal Transplantation (2002) European best practice guidelines for renal transplantation Section IV: Long-term management of the transplant recipient. IV.5.1. Cardiovascular risks. Cardiovascular disease after renal transplantation. *Nephrology, Dialysis and Transplantation*; **17** (Suppl 4): 24–5.

Human Tissue Authority website. Available at URL http://www.hta.gov.uk

Karlberg I, Nyberg G. (1995) Cost-effectiveness studies of renal transplantation. *International Journal of Technology Assessment in Health Care*; **11**: 611–22.

Laupacis A, Keown P, Pus N *et al.* (1996) A study of the quality of life and cost utility of renal transplantation. *Kidney International*; **50**: 235–42.

Murray JE, Merrill JP, Harrison JH. (1955) Renal homotransplantation in identical twins. *Surgical Forum VI* 432–6.

UK Transplant Support Service Authority. *National Protocols and Guidelines (renal)*. Available at URL http://www.uktransplant.org.uk/ukt/about_transplants/organ_allocation/kidney_(renal)/national_protocols_and_guidelines/national_protocols_and_guidelines.jsp

Wolfe RA, Ashby, VB, Milford EL *et al.* (1999) Comparison of mortality in all patients on dialysis awaiting transplantation, and recipients of a first cadaveric transplant. *New England Journal of Medicine*; **341**: 1725–30.

CHAPTER 12

The Organization of Services for People with Chronic Kidney Disease – a 21st Century Challenge

Donal O'Donoghue, John Feehally

OVERVIEW

- Between 22 and 57% of patients start dialysis without adequate preparation within the UK. This is often due to a failure to integrate care, such as in patients with diabetes.
- The National Service Framework for kidney disease identifies as markers of best practice in the pre-dialysis phase:
  - multi-professional care for at least one year before renal replacement therapy;
  - vascular access at least 6 months before haemodialysis;
  - pre-emptive transplant listing at a GFR of 15mL/min or 6 months before dialysis;
- 'Satellite' units that are available for the more stable haemodialysis patients are now more numerous, but despite this, the travelling time for many haemodialysis patients is still in excess of the 'standard' of less than 30 minutes.
- System re-design is required to address the challenges of providing equitable, efficient and high quality care to people with kidney disease.
- New methods of haemodialysis are emerging. In some units there are patients who are now taking a more independent role in managing their own haemodialysis. 'Home haemodialysis' is also being offered in a growing number of areas. This avoids the travel three times a week to and from the dialysis centre, and the option of overnight dialysis at home allows longer and possibly more efficient sessions.

Introduction

Renal medicine as a clinical speciality is a relative newcomer. Prior to the 1960s, when long-term renal replacement therapy first became available as a result of vascular access and transplant surgery, clinical care of people with kidney disease consisted of little more than observing progressive pathophysiology for which there was little treatment. Care of patients on renal replacement therapy now provides the major workload for renal teams, although nephrologists still have a significant role in the management of acute renal failure and in the investigation and treatment of a wide range of kidney diseases, which nowadays do not necessarily lead to renal failure.

Until the recent publication of the Renal National Service Framework (NSF) policy, initiatives focused exclusively on dialysis and transplantation. It is now recognized that the renal care pathway is much broader. A preventative dividend may be achieved if we had a better understanding of factors responsible for the initiation of renal injury and by the early detection and active management of progressive kidney disease.

There is now a clear appreciation of by how much the numbers of people affected by some degree of chronic kidney disease (CKD) are increasing (Box 12.1)– this has been labelled an 'epidemic' in some quarters. This large expansion in affected individuals has been fuelled both by global increases in obesity and type 2 diabetes mellitus (Table 12.1), and also by a better understanding of how to describe the earlier manifestations of CKD – in terms of microalbuminuria, and early reduction in renal function (GFR) (Box 12.2).

Box 12.1 **Key facts**

CKD
- >5% of population;
- co-morbidity: 90% HT, 40% CVD, 20% DM;
- Standard mortality rate (SMR) 36 in unreferred <60 years;
- optimal therapy 30%;
- potential savings in US $18–60 bn/10 years.

ERF
- increasing at 6–8% p.a.;
- acute uraemic emergencies 22–57%;
- pre-emptive transplant listing 3–54%;
- dialysis survival 1st year 75–93%;
- Cost £0.4 bn/year (2002/03) rising to >£0.8 bn/year (2010/11).

Table 12.1 The prevalence and incidence of chronic kidney disease and diabetes in several developed countries (in patients per million population)

Country	Prevalence	Incidence	Diabetic
USA	1390	334	148
Germany	918	174	62.6
Italy	835	137	23.3
Austria	769	130	44.2
Canada	761	143	45.8
Norway	756	92.3	11
Sweden	756	113.7	23.7
New Zealand	685	115	52
Netherlands	660	100	16
Australia	658	94	24.4
UK	626	101	18.1

Box 12.2 **Early detection of kidney disease**

Most patients with CKD will be detected by systematic surveillance – measuring eGFR in high risk groups
- hypertension;
- diabetes;
- cardiovascular disease including heart failure;
- patients receiving diuretics, ACE inhibitors, ARB, long-term NSAIDs and other nephrotoxic agents;
- black and minority ethnic populations;
- family history of renal disease.

Why?
- To minimize associated risks – especially cardiovascular morbidity.
- To minimize complications of CKD.
- To delay or prevent ERF.
- To avoid late referral.

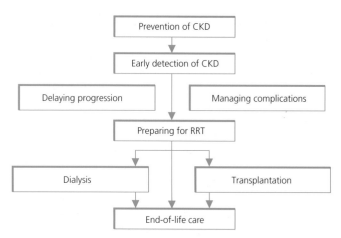

Figure 12.1 The kidney patient pathway.

Box 12.3 **The challenges facing renal healthcare**

- Integrating CKD management into other vascular disease programmes.
- Expansion of dialysis services.
- Increasing the number of kidney donors.
- Establishing supportive and palliative care for people with CKD.

The current model of service

Services for people with kidney disease in the UK originally developed in teaching hospitals, mostly alongside academic departments, but have over the last 20 years expanded into some district hospitals. Over that time the number of people on renal replacement therapy has more than quadrupled. Yet by international comparison, the UK lags significantly behind other developed countries in the provision of renal services. The renal community of care remains small, with only 78 main renal departments providing in-patient services. Twenty-three of these are combined with a transplant unit on-site. In the last decade, outreach clinics have been established in many district hospitals. Satellite units providing dialysis for stable patients are now much more numerous, and approaching half of all haemodialysis patients are now managed in these local units. Despite this growth, for the majority of patients the travelling time for haemodialysis, which is a thrice-weekly treatment, remains in excess of the standard of less than 30 minutes.

One of the major continuing challenges is the development of new renal services alongside the continued necessary expansion of existing dialysis and renal units. Changes in patterns of working to achieve this are both inevitable and increasingly desirable. Renal services need a stable commissioning and planning platform from which to respond to local needs.

Challenges for renal healthcare

The 'historical' centralized model of care is ill-equipped to manage the epidemic of chronic kidney disease and provide long-term support across the whole kidney patient pathway, much of which by definition will take place in a community setting (Fig 12.1). System redesign is likely to be required to address the challenges of providing equitable, timely, efficient and high quality care to people with kidney disease (Box 12.3). Although the number of consultant nephrologists has almost doubled in the last 10 years, and this growth continues, investment in education and training of the whole renal multi-professional team is required to provide a motivated, flexible and empowered workforce to meet the needs of these patients. Of the greatest importance is the understanding that community-based or primary care must play an increasingly important role in

this endeavour, complementing other groups. An integrated care plan, a central pillar of the Renal NSF, requires information systems that work across institutional, professional and geographic barriers. This can be achieved, but current realization is patchy across the UK and will require sustained investment and resources.

The roles of primary care

Inclusion of a CKD domain within the Quality and Outcomes Framework (QOF) of the General Medical Services (GMS) Contract from April 2006 has placed the emphasis for the detection of early kidney disease in primary care (Table 12.2). Establishing practice-based registers of CKD is the cornerstone of chronic disease management. The universal adoption in 2006 of the KDOQI (Kidney Dialysis Outcomes Quality Initiative) classification of the stages of CKD and the automatic reporting of estimated glomerular filtration rates (eGFR) by clinical chemistry laboratories now facilitate the creation of these registers. Those at risk of CKD have been defined by the Renal NSF.

Table 12.2 The chronic kidney disease (CKD) domain of Quality and Outcomes Framework (2006/7)

	Points	Payment stages
CKD1: A register of patients aged 18 years and over with CKD (stage 3–5 CKD)	6	
CKD2: Percentage of patients with a record of BP in the last 15 months	6	40–90%
CKD3: Percentage of patients with a BP of 140/85 or less	11	40–70%
CKD4: Percentage of patients who are treated with an ACE-I and ARB (unless a contraindication)	4	40–80%

See Fig. 12.2 for the situation in the average GP practice. From community-based research we know that the majority of those with moderate to severe CKD are already having serial serum creatinine measurements. Some of these are opportunistic, often during an intercurrent illness, whilst others are part of regular monitoring of people known to have hypertension, vascular disease or diabetes.

Recall of those on the *register* for *regular review*, the three Rs of chronic disease management, will enable a systematic approach to patient management to be implemented. The importance of vascular risk reduction in improving vascular and renal outcomes has already been emphasized in previous chapters.

There is an opportunity to integrate vascular care using the same GP-based systems for coronary heart disease, kidney disease, diabetes and stroke. However, the perception that kidney disease is complex, rare and always requires specialist care is inimical to such a holistic approach. Demystifying kidney disease and its management (one of the aims of this book) requires a shift in the paradigm from serum creatinine to eGFR, alongside the use of 'percentage kidney function' as the currency of kidney disease in the education of healthcare professionals and particularly in the empowerment of people with kidney disease (Fig. 12.3).

For the majority of those with kidney disease, an appreciation of their increased vascular risk, and inclusion of interventions to minimize this in their care plan, is required. A minority where the diagnosis is unclear, with features of progression (such as proteinuria, falling eGFR or uncontrolled hypertension) or with the complications of advanced chronic kidney disease, can benefit most from specialist care.

The recently published UK guidelines on the management of CKD provide referral templates. We know from the falling rates of coronary heart disease and cancer in many parts of the world that such a population-based systematic approach to care can be effective.

Planning for renal replacement therapy

Patients who arrive as 'crash landers' (with advanced CKD, but unknown to local renal services) requiring urgent unplanned dialysis, have poorer outcomes compared to those who have experienced educational programmes, been given the opportunity to make informed choices regarding renal replacement therapy modality, and who start dialysis in a planned fashion or receive a pre-emptive trans-

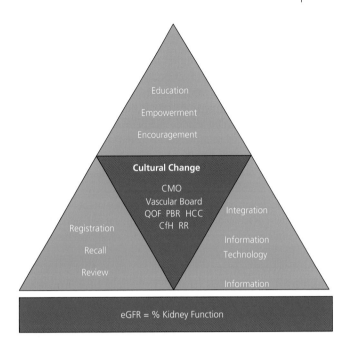

Figure 12.3 Demystifying and managing chronic renal disease. CfH: connecting for health; CMO: chief medical officer; HCC: health care commission; PBR: payment by results; QOF: Quality and Outcomes Framework, RR: renal registry.

plant (see Chapters 9–11). These 'crash' patients have twice the mortality and three times the length of hospitalization in their first year on dialysis. In the UK, depending on where patients live, between 22 and 57% of people start dialysis without this adequate preparation. In many cases, such as in people with diabetes, this almost certainly reflects a failure to integrate care. The Renal NSF identifies multi-professional care for at least one year, vascular access surgery 6 months before haemodialysis, and pre-emptive transplant listing at a GFR of 15 mL/min, or 6 months before dialysis, as markers of best practice in the pre-dialysis phase (Box 12.4).

Pre-dialysis services are under-developed. A recent survey found that an estimated number of 140 000 CKD patients were under the care of UK nephrologists but few units had access to the full complement of the recommended multi-skilled team. Counsellors and psychologists were the most commonly perceived shortages and the current provision of service was found to be patchy and variable.

Box 12.4 **Pre-dialysis care: NSF markers of good practice**

- Referral to a multi-skilled team, if possible at least one year before start of dialysis.
- Accelerated, intensive input from renal team for those who present late.
- People with ERF given information about all forms of treatment so that informed choice can be made.
- Patients put on transplant list within 6 months of their anticipated start of dialysis.
- Anaemia treated to maintain an adequate haemoglobin level.
- Management of cardiovascular risk factors and diabetes according to NSFs for CHD and diabetes.

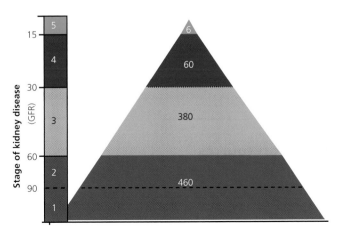

Figure 12.2 Chronic kidney disease in a typical GP practice of 10 000.

Dialysis and transplantation

Renal replacement therapy requires additional skills to pre-dialysis care. This includes catering for critically ill people with acute renal failure, those requiring intense immunosuppression and those with complex metabolic disarray. In contrast to the pre-dialysis care, however, we have high-quality activity and performance data for long-term dialysis and renal transplantation from the UK Renal Registry and UK Transplant. The UK Renal Registry has achieved universal coverage for all patients on renal replacement therapy in the UK, and has long-established robust audit arrangements that provide an ideal vehicle for continuous quality improvement of care. The challenge here is to ensure that the development of Connecting for Health builds on this expertise and provides additional functionality to extend the scope of comparative national audit.

The delivery of patient-centred care has always been a challenge which renal medicine has relished; renal units have many long-standing 'expert' patients who rightly understand the importance of excellent information and proper communication to assist their decision-making. This has now been taken one step further with Renal Patient View, a unique system developed by the renal community that allows patients direct personal web-based access to appropriate information directly downloaded from clinical information systems in renal units.

Transplantation is the best form of renal replacement therapy for those that are suitable – which is up to 40% of those receiving dialysis. Figure 12.4 shows that for the first time in many years transplantation now represents less than 50% of the total population receiving renal replacement therapy. Transplantation, particularly live donation, has unique challenges which include paying attention to societal views, increasing public awareness and garnering its support. Transplantation care is much wider than the kidney engraftment operation itself, and the periods immediately before and after this. It includes recipient preparation, donor care, relationships with critical care colleagues and long-term post-transplant care with its elements of increased vascular risk, complications of CKD, and unusual pattern of malignancy risks.

Independent sector treatment centres

One aspect of renal care, maintenance of thrice weekly out-patient haemodialysis, is potentially suitable for a differing model of health-

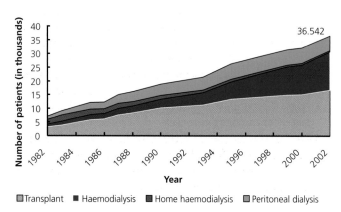

Figure 12.4 Renal replacement therapy modalities.

Box 12.5 **Criteria for supportive care in CKD**

At least two of the indicators below:
- CKD stage 5 (eGFR < 15 mL/min).
- Frail individuals at CKD stage 4 (eGFR 15–25 mL/min).
- Patients thought to be in the last year of life by the care team – the 'surprise question'.
- Patients choosing the no dialysis option, discontinuing dialysis or opting not to restart dialysis if their transplant is failing.
- Difficult physical symptoms (e.g. anorexia, nausea, pruritus, reduced function status, intractable fluid overload) or psychological symptoms despite optimal tolerated therapy.

care delivery such as the independent sector treatment centres (ISTCs) which are now being vigorously adopted as government policy. The concept is not new to renal care. There is a 20-year experience in this country of offering maintenance dialysis in satellite dialysis facilities built and maintained by (private) specialist dialysis companies. Many of the issues which concern observers of the ISTC innovation, including achieving proper quality control, ensuring seamless transition between the independent sector and the NHS when required, proper information transfer, uniform standards of care – have all long been resolved by NHS renal units working with their commercial partners in such facilities. Experience dictates that with open tendering, private providers sometimes, but not always, win contracts for such satellite units and can offer significant value for money.

Supportive and palliative care in CKD

Chronic kidney disease is a disease of the elderly and is associated with a range of co-morbidities (Box 12.5). Many patients elect not to have dialysis as their long-term prognosis and quality of life independent of CKD is poor. This important area is explored more fully in Chapter 9.

Conclusion

Chronic kidney disease is a long-term condition, whose frequency is increasing. Provision of dialysis facilities is very expensive. Prevention makes huge societal, medical and financial sense. Part of CKD care will occur in an acute setting and hospitals are likely to remain the major provider of renal replacement therapy programmes. But to achieve the integrated care necessary for an efficient high quality service envisioned by the Renal NSF, commissioning of pathways of care will be necessary so that resources can be made available at the right part of the pathway at the right time.

Further resources

NSF Parts 1 and 2, http://www.dh.gov.uk/PolicyAndGuidance/HealthAndSocialCareTopics/Renal/fs/en
Renal Registry and Renal Registry Report, http://www.renalreg.com
The Renal Association, http://www.renal.org/ and http://www.renal.org/eGFR/eguide.html
UK Transplant, http://www.uktransplant.org.uk

APPENDIX 1

Glossary of Renal Terms and Conditions

David Goldsmith

This section provides an easy quick reference guide for those 'diagnoses' that so often appear in discharge summaries from renal teams to GPs and other non-nephrology consultants. We provide only the bare bones of a description and the key things to know. Anyone interested in more detailed learning can use one or more of the many online resources to which we have provided links..

Alport's syndrome

See Chapter 8, p. 43.

Anti-GBM (Goodpasture's) disease

This is a very rare disease which is a small vessel vasculitis involving the renal capillaries (presenting as acute renal failure/RPGN) and sometimes the pulmonary capillaries (presenting as acute severe pulmonary haemorrhage).

Diagnosis is made on clinical grounds, and backed up by changes in chest X-ray, lung function testing, circulating anti-GBM antibodies (performed by specialized immunology laboratories) and renal biopsy.

Typically this is an aggressive one-shot illness seen in younger patients, and results in rapid renal failure or fatal lung bleeding. Aggressive immunosuppression including plasma exchange can reduce the risk from lung haemorrhage, but rarely can severe/permanent renal failure be prevented.

Autosomal dominant polycystic kidney disease (ADPKD)

See Chapter 6, p. 30.

Diabetic nephropathy (DN)

Diabetes (type 1 and 2) constitutes the commonest current cause of established renal failure in the industrialized world. Type 2 diabetes is rapidly increasing in prevalence and, although often a disease of middle to old age, is occurring more frequently in younger age-groups as global obesity increases.

In about a third of patients, renal involvement can occur, usually after 10–20 years of diabetes (diabetic nephropathy is a small vessel complication, such as sensorimotor/autonomic neuropathy, retinopathy and small arteriolar disease). The first sign of renal involvement by diabetic nephropathy is microalbuminuria (MAU) (see Chapters 1–3). Early treatment with ACEI and ARB, to lower blood pressure and reduce MAU, can abort the otherwise inevitable progression to overt proteinuria and renal functional decline.

It is of the greatest importance that all patients with diabetes have annual urine testing for the presence of MAU, and have meticulous attention paid to overall metabolic control, dyslipidaemia and blood pressure. Cardiovascular disease is very common in all diabetics, the more so in those with any degree of renal disease.

Focal segmental glomerulosclerosis (FSGS)

FSGS is a diagnostic term for a clinico-pathological syndrome with multiple aetiologies. FSGS is becoming a more common renal condition, and is the commonest renal lesion (excepting diabetic nephropathy) in black patients. It can be idiopathic, or secondary to other renal pathologies and lesions.

Presentation can be at any age, and is usually with isolated proteinuria or more commonly nephrotic syndrome. Hypertension and renal impairment are common.

Diagnosis is by means of renal biopsy. Treatment can be effected by ACEI and ARBs to reduce proteinuria, and blood pressure. Long courses of prednisolone, or other immunosuppressants, can help in selected cases.

Glomerulonephritis (Gn)

Glomerulonephritis (see Chapter 8, p.44) covers glomerular disease, is often (but not always) inflammatory in nature, and can be primary or secondary to another systemic illness (e.g. lupus).

Gn causes raised blood pressure, oedema, renal impairment, microscopic haematuria (sometimes macroscopic) and significant proteinuria (PCR > 100). There may also be signs relating to any underlying inflammatory, degenerative, metabolic or other systemic processes (e.g. vasculitic rash).

Depending on the type of Gn, the age of the patient and the extent of reversible versus irreversible renal damage, there can be therapies to retard or regress the Gn. Acute renal vasculitis can be effectively treated with potent immunosuppressives.

IgA disease and Henoch–Schönlein purpura (HSP)

IgA-nephropathy (IgA-N) is a form of primary Gn, and is the commonest form of primary Gn in most parts of the world. It occurs in all age groups, but is most common in younger people (children and adolescents). In younger patients, recurrent macroscopic haematuria, and intermittent or persistent proteinuria, with hypertension, are the commonest presentations. Exacerbations of symptoms often occur with febrile illnesses, or upper respiratory tract infection/tonsillitis. In older subjects, the signs are less dramatic as macroscopic haematuria is rarer. IgA-N is a significant cause of isolated microscopic haematuria (see Chapter 1, p. 2).

Particularly in children and adolescents, but more rarely in adults, there can be a symptom complex of vasculitic rash on extensor surfaces, arthralgia, gastro-intestinal pain and haemorrhage (e.g. rectal bleeding) with acute IgA-N. This is known as HSP. Anti-pyretics, analgesics and sometimes steroids can help the systemic features.

The diagnosis can only be made by renal biopsy, and this is essential as other forms of glomerular disease can present in similar ways. Treating proteinuria and hypertension using ACEI and ARBs is practical and sensible. There is no consensus about the utility of more specific therapies; trials of prednisolone, plus more potent immunosuppression, fish oils, and other interventions e.g. tonsillectomy, have failed to resolve this matter.

Interstitial nephritis

Acute interstitial nephritis (AIN) is an acute, sometimes reversible, inflammatory disease diagnosed after renal biopsy. It is a relatively common cause of renal dysfunction (15% of acute renal failure in some series). It can occur at any age, though is rarer in children. Drugs – antibiotics, non-steroidals, allopurinol, diuretics – are frequent causes of AIN, which can also be idiopathic, secondary to Chinese herbs, other nephrotoxins, infections, collagen vascular disease, and malignancy.

Presentation is with oliguria in many cases, in the context of renal impairment, which can progress rapidly. Where an allergic reaction to a drug is the reason for AIN, there can be fever, rash, arthralgia, eosinophilia-eosinophiluria, sterile pyuria. Conventional urinalysis for blood and protein can be bland.

Stopping any potentially responsible drugs, and a short course of prednisolone, are typical interventions. Recovery is usual, though not universal, and some residual renal impairment due to renal interstitial fibrosis secondary to the inflammation is common.

Lupus nephritis (LN)

Systemic lupus can affect the kidney. In rare cases the only manifestation of lupus is renal disease. Involvement can range from low-grade proteinuria/microscopic haematuria, through nephrotic syndrome, to fulminant acute renal failure. Systemic lupus classically presents in pre-menopausal women, with hair loss, mouth ulcers, skin rash, and arthralgia. More rarely, venous thrombotic episodes may herald anti-phospholipid syndrome, either in isolation or as part of classical SLE.

Renal lupus is diagnosed in the clinical context of SLE, with positive autoantibodies and after a renal biopsy, which is necessary to delineate the extent and severity of renal involvement. Treatment involves a combination of blood pressure reduction, possible anti-coagulation (if anti-phospholipid positive) and immunosuppression (as above).

Membranous nephropathy (MN)

MN is a relatively common renal lesion, and one of the leading causes of primary glomerular disease. It is found in subjects of all ages, with a peak incidence in middle to old age. It is more common in men than women. Presentation is typically with isolated proteinuria, nephrotic syndrome, hypertension and renal impairment.

MN can be idiopathic, or secondary to underlying malignancy (lung, colon, other), systemic infection, HIV, hepatitis B or C, SLE, or drugs such as gold, penicillamine, non-steroidals and others.

ACEI and ARB are used for raised blood pressure and proteinuria. Persistent nephrotic syndrome and progressive renal impairment are indications for immunosuppression, with prednisolone and other agents such as chlorambucil, cyclophosphamide or ciclosporin.

Minimal change nephropathy (MCN)

MCN is the commonest cause of nephrotic syndrome in children (70–90%) and younger adults (50%). It is diagnosed more rarely in older subjects. It is a histological diagnosis, reached after renal biopsy. In children (see Chapter 8, p.43) it is usual to treat acute-onset nephrotic syndrome with steroids, but in adults a renal biopsy is usually performed before treatment, as the differential diagnosis is wider. Primary MN is by far the most common, but secondary MN is known in association with viral infection, HIV, drug use and malignancy.

Presentation is typically with acute onset nephrotic syndrome (see Chapter 4). Oedema can be prodigious, and pleural and pericardial effusions and ascites can be severe.

Treatment is with oral prednisolone for many weeks (typically 3 months). Response rates are best in children and young adults. Relapse is not usual, though some patients relapse in a predictable fashion as steroid doses fall. Acute infections can also precipitate relapse. Other drugs, in steroid-insensitive, or steroid-dependent subjects, may be needed..

Myeloma, amyloid and the kidney

Renal involvement by myeloma is quite common. This can be as a result of hypercalcaemia, hyperuricaemia, cast nephropathy, interstitial nephritis and direct infiltration by plasma cells. The presentation can be proteinuria, hypertension and renal impairment.

Immunocyte (AL) and reactive (AA) amyloid can affect the kidney, with the usual presentation being isolated proteinuria, more typically nephrotic syndrome.

Treatment of the underlying condition leading to myeloma or amyloidosis is the only specific intervention. Renal impairment can limit chemotherapy options.

Nephrotic syndrome

See Chapter 4

Pyelonephritis

Acute pyelonephritis (AP; see Chapter 6) is infection of the renal parenchyma caused by bacterial infection ascending the urinary tract from the bladder.

Like acute cystitis, AP is much more common in women than men. Risk factors include structural abnormalities of the urinary tract, pregnancy, diabetes, asymptomatic bacteriuria, urinary tract instrumentation and sexual intercourse. In men AP is more often seen over the age of 40, with prostatic disease and renal stones being the commonest underlying reasons.

The commonest micro-organisms are *Escherichia coli*, *Proteus*, *Pseudonomas*, and *Klebsiella* spp.

Patients usually present with fever, rigors, loin pain and lower urinary tract symptoms. Loin pain and tenderness can be severe. There can be septicaemic shock where there is obstruction or immunosuppression. Leucocytosis, raised CRP, urine and blood cultures can all aid diagnosis. Renal ultrasound usually shows an enlarged kidney.

Treatment is with appropriate antibiotics, administered intravenously in severe cases. Obstruction should be relieved.

Renal (ANCA positive) vasculitis

Vasculitis can involve large blood vessels, and smaller ones. Only small vessel vasculitis commonly involves the kidney – this involvement can be anything from low-grade proteinuria/microscopic haematuria, through nephrotic syndrome, to fulminant acute renal failure (a synonym of which is RPGN or rapidly progressive glomerulonephritis).

This is characteristically a disease of middle-aged to elderly patients, though it can occur in children. Presentation can be 'renal only' i.e. no systemic vasculitis features clinically, to multiple organ/system involvement. Joint pains, myalgia, skin rash, iritis, uveitis,

general malaise, anorexia and weight loss can accompany any renal manifestations.

One important association is pulmonary–renal syndromes. The lung and the kidney can be involved in vasculitis in Goodpasture's syndrome (acute pulmonary haemorrhage), Wegener's granulomatosis (haemoptysis, breathlessness, lung nodules on chest x-ray or CT, and often deafness and nasal blockage and epistaxis), Churg-Strauss syndrome (with asthma and eosinophilia) and lupus.

Diagnosis comes from correctly interpreting the multi-system features. Anaemia, raised white count and thrombocytosis are common. The ESR and CRP are raised. More specific tests include anti-neutrophil cytoplasmic antibodies (ANCA).

Treatment with potent immunosuppressives (prednisolone, azathioprine, mycophenolate mofetil, cyclophosphamide, plasma exchange) can be very effective, especially if the diagnosis is made promptly, before life-threatening complications ensue. Without treatment, these diseases are often fatal.

Renovascular disease

See Chapter 5.

Thin membrane nephropathy (TMN)

Persistent microscopic haematuria (see Chapter 1) is seen in around 3–5% of the UK population. TMN is responsible for about 20–40% of this. TMN can be sporadic, or more rarely, familial. Diagnosis is made by electron microscopy of a renal biopsy specimen (measuring the width of the glomerular basement membrane, which is reduced in TMN).

This condition is usually asymptomatic, and is diagnosed on medical screening where this includes urinalysis (e.g. health, insurance medicals). Onset can be in childhood. Haematuria in TMN can be microscopic or macroscopic, intermittent or persistent. Sometimes the macroscopic haematuria can be painful, and very rarely, heavy enough to cause temporary ureteric or bladder obstruction. Prognosis is usually excellent

APPENDIX 2

Anaemia Management in Chronic Kidney Disease

Penny Ackland

Anaemia contributes significantly to the heavy symptom burden of chronic kidney disease (CKD), its presence having a major impact on the quality of life and physical capacity of the patient. It becomes more prevalent the more advanced the stage of CKD (1% of people with an eGFR of 60 mL/min, 9% of people with an eGFR of 30 ml/min, and 33% of people with an eGFR of 15 ml/min are anaemic). The overall incidence of anaemia in CKD stages 3 to 5 is 12%.

The anaemia of CKD is normochromic and normocytic in nature. The causes are often multifactorial, but by far the main contribution is the reduced erythropoietic activity caused by iron deficiency, erythropoietin deficiency, or both. Other minor causes may also contribute to the anaemia of CKD.

The NICE guideline on *Anaemia Management in People with Chronic Kidney Disease* suggests consideration of treating the anaemia in adults/children over the age of 2 years, when the haemoglobin is ≤ 11 g/dL. The treatment will depend on the underlying cause. Deficiencies of both iron and erythropoietin can be corrected by replacement therapy, and thus the relative contribution of theses causes should be ascertained.

Laboratory parameters, which may be used for detecting iron deficiency, include the serum ferritin level, transferrin saturation, and percentage of hypochromic red cells. A serum ferritin level of < 100 μg/L is diagnostic of iron deficiency anaemia (IDA) in stage 5 CKD, and may indicate IDA in stages 3 and 4 CKD. Even when the serum ferritin is greater than 100 μg/L, functional iron deficiency may still be present if the transferrin saturation is < 20% or the percentage hypochromic red cells is > 6%. Diagnostic cut-off values for serum ferritin as an indicator of iron deficiency are very different in the CKD population (due to the inherent chronic inflammatory state) compared to the general population.

If severe iron deficiency is present (e.g. serum ferritin < 30 μg/L), then it is important to consider possible blood loss as a contributory cause to the anaemia.

Blood loss may be overt or occult, and although overt blood loss may be ascertained from careful history taking, occult gastrointestinal blood loss may be present in many CKD patients who have an increased bleeding tendency due to platelet defects associated with uraemia, aspirin therapy, etc. Furthermore, additional factors causing blood loss in stage 5 CKD patients on dialysis include entrapment of red cells in the dialyser, and use of heparin during the dialysis session. Upper gastrointestinal endoscopy and/or colonoscopy may be indicated if occult gastrointestinal blood loss is suspected.

If blood loss has been excluded as far as is possible, then iron deficiency should be corrected by administration of supplemental iron. Oral iron can be given, but unfortunately in many CKD patients iron absorption is impaired, and this is particularly evident in patients with advanced renal impairment. Side-effects are common, and compliance with treatment may be low. Many CKD patients therefore require intravenous iron. Iron correction should aim to keep the serum ferritin level above 200 μg/L. Further iron administration should not be administered if the serum ferritin is above 500 μg/L and the aim should be to keep the ferritin level below 800 μg/L.

CKD patients who are anaemic but iron-replete should be considered for erythropoiesis-stimulating agent (ESA) therapy. Treatment with ESAs should be offered to all who are likely to benefit in terms of quality of life and physical function. Age alone should not be a determinant for the use of such therapy. The aim should be to maintain stable haemoglobin levels between 10.5 and 12.5 g/dL. This is clearly lower that normal for healthy individuals, but, apart from quality of life, there is no evidence that aiming for complete correction of anaemia is of benefit in this patient population, and there may even be increased risk of harm. The aspirational target haemoglobin range should be achieved by adjusting treatment, typically when the Hb rises above 12 g/dL or falls below 11 g/dL. Patient preferences, symptoms, and co-morbidities may also impact on the appropriate target haemoglobin range.

In patients who are showing a poor response to treatment, one should:

- evaluate concordance;
- measure reticulocyte count – if high, consider blood loss and haemolysis;
- exclude other causes of anaemia (Box A2.1);
- exclude intercurrent illness;
- exclude chronic blood loss;
- consider bone marrow examination.

Box A2.1 **Other possible causes of anaemia in CKD**

- Chronic blood loss
- Iron deficiency
- Vitamin B_{12} or folate deficiency
- Hypothyroidism
- Chronic infection or inflammation
- Hyperparathyroidism
- Aluminium toxicity
- Malignancy
- Haemolysis
- Bone marrow infiltration
- Pure red cell aplasia

Chronic Kidney Disease and Drug Prescribing

Douglas Maclean, Satish Jaywardene

Many commonly prescribed medicines are metabolized or excreted by the kidney. Impaired renal function can alter drug behaviour in the body, including:

- reduction in renal excretion of a drug or its metabolites may lead to potential accumulation and associated toxic effects;
- the build-up of uraemic toxins may be associated with alterations in behaviour of drugs within the body;
- alterations in absorption of medicines, e.g. reduction in the absorption of furosemide following oral administration in patients with visceral oedema;
- changes in sensitivity of the body to some drugs even if elimination is not compromised, e.g. opiates increase cerebral sensitivity;
- tissue distribution of certain drugs may alter as a consequence of accumulation of body water and, or, reduced renal clearance of uraemic toxins, e.g. antibiotics including gentamicin, amikacin;
- binding of drugs to proteins in the blood may be reduced in nephrotic syndrome, e.g. flucloxacillin, phenytoin and sodium valproate, with increased risk of toxicity.

Many of these factors have implications for drug prescribing in patients with compromised renal function, in terms of the choice of drug and the dose prescribed. Failure to consider these may place such patients at increased risk of drug-related adverse effects, including renal toxicity.

Drugs with a narrow therapeutic window, e.g. anti-arrhythmics such as disopyramide, flecainide, lidocaine nadolol, sotalol, in addition to other agents including aciclovir, clozapine, digoxin, ethambutol, lithium and methotrexate, dosing regimens based on glomerular filtration (mainly creatinine clearance estimates) should be used. For many of these drugs, whose efficacy and toxicity are closely related to serum concentrations, dosing should be determined both in terms of clinical response and quantifiable measures, e.g. INR for patients undergoing treatment with warfarin. Serum levels can also be useful to aid drug dosing, allowing optimization of clinical effect with minimization of toxicity. See also Table A3.1.

Drugs that may impair kidney function

Drugs can be nephrotoxic through a variety of pathophysiological mechanisms, including pre-renal hypoperfusion (e.g. captopril), glomerulopathy (e.g. penicillamine, gold), allergic interstitial nephritis (e.g. antibiotics, proton pump inhibitors), direct tubular toxicity (e.g. aminoglycosides, high dose rosuvastatin) and tubular obstruction (e.g. sulphonamides). Patient factors such as dehydra-

tion, sepsis, pre-existing heart failure and concomitant drug therapy (e.g. non-steroidal anti-inflammatory drugs; NSAIDs, diuretics and ACE inhibitors/angiotensin II receptor blockers) will increase inherent risk of drug-related toxicity.

Drugs affected by pre-existing kidney disease

The renal excretion of many drugs may depend on the glomerular filtration rate, a balance between secretion and reabsorption of drugs in the renal tubules or renal drug metabolism, e.g. insulin and interferons. When GFR is reduced in renal disease, the clearance of drugs eliminated by the kidney is decreased and the plasma half-life is prolonged, e.g. aciclovir, opiates, digoxin, sotalol.

Drug prescribing in renal impairment

Special care is required when interpreting advice on dose adjustment based on creatinine clearance (e.g. calculated from the Cockcroft and Gault formula) because renal function is increasingly being reported on the basis of estimated glomerular filtration rate (eGFR) normalized to a body surface area of $1.73\,m^2$ and derived from the MDRD (Modification of Diet in Renal Disease) formula. **The two measures of renal function cannot be used interchangeably.**

Pain management in patients with chronic kidney disease

Pain is one of the most common symptoms experienced by patients with chronic kidney disease; it impairs their quality of life and is under-treated.

The World Health Organization (WHO) three-step analgesic ladder is a helpful aid to guidance on pain management in these patients (Figure A3.1).

Paracetamol 500 mg to 1 g four times a day given regularly should be considered for mild pain associated with CKD. Paracetamol is available in various dose formulations, including liquid, tablets and soluble tablets and suppositories. No dosage modification is required for any degree of impaired renal function.

Non-steroidal anti-inflammatory drugs

All non-steroidal anti-inflammatory drugs (NSAIDs) should be avoided in patients with mild to moderate impaired renal function. They can further dramatically accelerate the rate of decline of renal function. Patients may also be predisposed to uraemic gastritis and

Table A3.1 Commonly prescribed anti-infective drugs in adults with pre-existing chronic kidney disease

Drug	Normal dose	Dose for impaired renal function and creatinine clearance
Aciclovir	Herpes Zoster: 800 mg five times a day Herpes Simplex: 200 mg five times a day or 400 mg five times a day in immunosuppressed patients	Herpes Zoster: 10–25 mL/min 800 mg every 8 hours or < 10 mL/min 800 mg every 12 hours Herpes Simplex: < 10 mL/min 200 mg every 12 hours or 400 mg every 12 hours in immunosuppressed patients
Cefaclor	250 mg every 8 hours	< 10 mL/min 125–250 mg every 8 hours
Cefadroxil	500 mg–1 g every 12–24 hours	< 10 mL/min 500 mg–1 g every 24–48 hours
Cephalexin	250 mg every 6 hours or 500 mg every 8–12 hours Recurrent UTI prophylaxis: 125 mg every night	10–20 mL/min 500 mg every 8–12 hours
Cefradine	250–500 mg every 6 hours or 500 mg–1 g every 12 hours	< 10 mL/min 250 mg every 6 hours
Ciprofloxacin	250–750 mg every 12 hours	< 10–20 mL/min half normal dose every 12 hours
Clarithromycin	250–500 mg every 12 hours	10–20 mL/min 250–500 mg every 12–24 hours < 10 mL/min 250 mg every 12–24 hours
Co-Amoxiclav	375–675 mg every 8 hours	< 10 mL/min 375 mg 8–12 hourly
Co-Trimoxazole	960 mg every 12 hours	15–30 mL/min 480 mg every 12 hours
Erythromycin	250–500 mg every 6 hours or 500 mg–1 g every 12 hours	< 10 mL/min: total daily dose < 1.5 g
Famciclovir	Herpes Zoster: 250 mg every eight hours First genital herpes infection: 250 mg every 8 hours Acute recurrent genital herpes: 125 mg every 12 hours	30–60 mL/min for Herpes Zoster and first genital herpes infection, 250 mg every 12 hours 10–30 mL/min for Herpes Zoster and first episode of genital herpes, 250 mg every 24 hours. Recurrent genital herpes: 125 mg every 24 hours < 10 mL/min
Nitrofurantoin	50–100 mg every 6 hours	< 50 mL/min contra-indicated as adequate urinary concentrations are not achieved
Ofloxacin	200–400 mg every 12 hours	Normal loading dose, then reduce to 100 mg every 24 hours
Terbinafine	250 mg every 24 hours	125 mg every 24 hours
Tetracyclines	250–500 mg every 6 hours	< 250–500 mg every 24 hours Will artificially increase serum creatinine so caution with use (doxycycline and minocycline are preferred)
Trimethoprim	200 mg every 12 hours	15–25 mL/min. Dose as in normal renal function for 3 days then 100 mg twice daily Will artificially increase serum creatinine so caution with use
Valaciclovir	Herpes Simplex: 500 mg every 12 hours Herpes Zoster: 1 g every 8 hours	15–30 mL/min, Herpes Simplex doses as in normal renal function Herpes Zoster: 1 g every 12–24 hours < 15 mL/min Herpes simplex, 500 mg daily Herpes Zoster: 500 mg–1 g every 24 hours

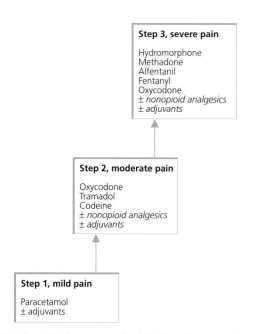

Figure A3.1 The WHO three-step analgesic ladder. Adjuvant analgesics are added to enhance analgesia such as steroids for pain from bone metastases. Adjuvants also includes medication such as anticonvulsants for neuropathic pain e.g. gabapentin, pregabalin and anti-depressants, e.g. amitriptyline, fluoxetine. Adapted from Barakzoy, A.S. and Moss, A.H. (2006) *Journal of the American Society of Nephrology*; **17**: 3198–203.

gastro-intestinal bleeding.

Cyclo-oxygenase inhibitors (COX-1) inhibitors include diclofenac, ibuprofen, mefenamic acid, naproxen, indomethacin and sulindac (a pro-drug which must be converted into its active form by the kidneys).

COX-2 inhibitors such as celecoxib and meloxicam, although believed to cause fewer adverse gastro-intestinal effects, should be prescribed with caution in these patients.

In established renal failure, non-steroidal drugs can be prescribed for patients where the clinical benefits outweigh the risks, usually in conjunction with gastro-protectant agents such as H2 receptor antagonists, e.g. cimetidine or ranitidine, or non-renally-cleared proton pump inhibitors including omeprazole.

Other analgesic options are shown in Table A3.2.

Parenteral diamorphine or morphine, especially if intravenous, should be administered with extreme caution in patients with compromised renal function as active metabolites that are renally excreted can accumulate. Diamorphine and morphine should only be prescribed when the therapeutic benefits clearly outweigh the clinical risks. It should be borne in mind that intravenous, intramuscular and subcutaneous doses of either diamorphine or morphine are not equipotent in terms of analgesic potency. If either of these drugs is to be administered, it should be commenced at the lowest doses available and reviewed regularly.

Table A3.2 Other analgesic options

Drug	Normal dose range	Modified dosing range for compromised renal function (creatinine clearance: mL/min)
Codeine phosphate	30–60 mg up to four times a day	20–50 mL/min dose as in normal renal function 10–20 mL/min 75% of normal dose < 10 mL/min 50% of normal dose
Tramadol	Oral 50–100 mg at intervals of not less than 4 hours. Maximum 600 mg daily. Parenterally intravenously or intramuscularly (severe uraemia can be associated with increased risks of haematoma formation and should possibly be avoided). 50–100 mg hourly to a total daily dose of 600 mg	20–50 mL/min dose as in normal renal function 10–20 mL/min, 50–100 mg every 12 hours < 10 mL/min 50 mg every 12 hours
Oxycodone	5 mg every 4–6 hours to a maximum daily dose of 400 mg. Modified release capsules can be administered initially at a dose of 10 mg every 12 hours titrating gradually upwards to 200 mg 12 hourly	An approach that may be adopted is to prescribe only the normal release capsules, extending the dose interval as long as may be tolerated. In patients with creatinine clearance < 10 mL/min oxycodone should be used with caution.
Fentanyl	50–200 μg by subcutaneous injection then 50 μg as required. Topical formulations of fentanyl includes lozenges and transdermal patches. Specialist advice should be sought for its use.	20–50 mL/min dose as in normal renal function 10–20 mL/min, 75% of normal dose < 10 mL/min, 50% of normal, titrate according to individual patient's response
Methadone	Methadone is a potent opioid analgesic which can be administered orally in doses of 5–10 mg every 6 to 8 hours	In patients with creatinine clearance < 10 mL/min the dose of methadone should be reduced by approximately 50% and titrated according to response
Hydromorphone	A potent opioid analgesic which can be commenced at doses of 1.3 mg every 4 hours increasing the dose as required. Sustained release capsules containing 2 and 4 mg are available. Initial starting doses with sustained release 2–4 mg every 12 hours. Specialist advice should be sought for its use.	Dose reductions may be required in patients with established renal failure, the metabolites of hydromorphone being eliminated by renal mechanisms

Table A3.3 Commonly prescribed drugs

Drug	Usual dose	Notes
Sodium bicarbonate	500 mg–2 g thrice daily	Used to treat the acidosis of renal failure Also helps lower serum potassium levels
ACE inhibitor/Angiotensin II receptor blocker	Depending upon formulation used	Used to reduce blood pressure and proteinuria Essential to check renal function and potassium 10–14 days following initiation
Calcium-based phosphate binders (calcium carbonate or calcium acetate)	Depending upon formulation used	Taken with meals to bind phosphate Dose adjusted according to phosphate and calcium levels
Non calcium-based phosphate binders (sevelamer or aluminium hydroxide)	Depending upon formulation used	Taken with meals to bind phosphate Dose adjusted according to phosphate levels Used in those who are hypercalcaemic
Iron (iron–sucrose; Venofer®)	100–200 mg intravenously. Frequency depends upon ferritin and haemoglobin level	Given to anaemic patients who are iron deficient
Erythropoietin stimulating agents (ESAs) (darbepoetin-alfa, epoetin-alfa, epoetin-beta)	Dose and frequency depends upon formulation and haemoglobin level	For management of anaemia associated with renal impairment ESAs are usually given subcutaneously
Alfacalcidol	Usually 0.25 μg once daily	Is a vitamin D analogue For the treatment of secondary hyperparathyroidism
N-acetyl cysteine	600 mg twice daily (4 doses)	Used for the prevention of contrast nephrotoxicity

Prescribing for patients with CKD/ERF

Table A3.3 shows a list of drugs, which are commonly prescribed in those patients with CKD. They are used especially in those with stages 3, 4 and 5 kidney disease. They are used to treat the symptoms and clinical sequelae of chronic kidney disease/established renal failure.

Further resources

Ashley C, Curie A. (eds) (2003) *The Renal Drug Handbook,* 2nd edn. Radcliffe Medical Press, Oxford.

Barakzoy AS, Moss AH. (2006) Efficacy of the World Health Organisation Analgesic Ladder to treat pain in end-stage renal disease. *J Am Soc Nephrol*; **17**: 3198–203.

Mehta, D (ed.) (2006) *British National Formulary 52*; Pharmaceutical Press, London.

Index

Note: page numbers in *italics* refer to figures, tables and boxes